Counselling for Loss and Bereavement

Counselling
for
Loss and Bereavement

VERENA TSCHUDIN
BSc (Hons) MA RGN RM DipCouns

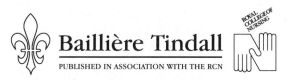

Baillière Tindall
PUBLISHED IN ASSOCIATION WITH THE RCN

London · Philadelphia · Toronto
Sydney · Tokyo

Baillière Tindall   24-28 Oval Road
London NW1 7DX

The Curtis Center
Independence Square West
Philadelphia, PA 19106-3399, USA

Harcourt Brace & Company
55 Horner Avenue
Toronto, Ontario, M8Z 4X6, Canada

Harcourt Brace & Company, Australia
30-52 Smidmore Street
Marrickville
NSW 2204, Australia

Harcourt Brace & Company, Japan
Ichibancho Central Building
22-1 Ichibancho
Chiyoda-ku, Tokyo 102, Japan

A catalogue record for this book is available from the British
Library

ISBN 0-7020-2131-8

Typeset by Photo-graphics, Honiton, Devon
Printed and bound in Great Britain by WBC Book Manufacturers
Ltd, Bridgend, Mid Glamorgan

Contents

....

....

Acknowledgements

I would like to thank all those who shared their stories with me. In every story some details have been changed in order to protect the persons concerned.

Special thanks go to those who wrote their stories.

The writer of 'Christmas puddings' could not be contacted and I would therefore like to thank her here.

My thanks also go to the person who suggested that this book should be written. Particular thanks go to Sarah James, Karen Gilmour, and all the staff at Baillière Tindall, for their friendship and constant support.

Preface

....

Throughout my writing career I have always felt happier when I worked on a text whose subject I had chosen myself. It felt more to be 'me' then, rather than writing to a request. So I was surprised when the request came for writing this present book. I had not thought of writing on the subject of counselling for loss and bereavement, but on reflection I wondered why I had never thought about it, because this reflected so obviously my counselling, and also my own personal experience.

I have learned in recent years that there are times of happiness and times of sorrow, times for receiving and times for giving, times for hanging on and times for letting go. In writing about loss I seem to be focusing on sorrow and grief and perhaps on letting go; yet by writing I am focusing on creativity, new understanding and receiving. This simply shows that the opposites are only illusions; in truth they are just like the two sides of a single coin.

I have always been grateful to my parents for letting my sister and me see a great-aunt after her death and go to the funeral. I was perhaps ten years old, and the sight of her in the coffin was not shocking, but somehow quite natural. This was the first significant loss in my life.

I was into my twenties when three of my grandparents died, and later I was able to nurse my dying grandfather for a few nights.

The really significant deaths happened later: at a particularly difficult time, while we were working in Jerusalem, the person who supported me most was killed by a bomb; my father died of a heart attack; a very special friend died abroad, and alone; an old man, who had become a client through the bereavement service I belonged to, died while I visited him in hospital.

But it is not only deaths which have been important. On the contrary, losses of other kinds have perhaps shaped me just as much as the loss of people. I have often wondered what I would say to a nurse who was conducting an interview on a hospital admission, and who might ask me what my significant losses were in my life. Would I tell that nurse that it was the loss of youth, of health, of dearly held values and beliefs, of certainties, of economic security, which shaped me most? And would I need to be specific about these losses? Would it help this nurse to care better for me if she or he knew of these things? Would it help me to have told them to a stranger? From experience I know how important it is to share something important when the moment is right. At that moment the other is no longer a stranger, but the significant other, in the full meaning of that expression.

My losses were and are enormously important, but they are not the sort of losses which can easily be seen and listed. Yet they have shaped me and made me what I am today. I have coped with them – more or less, as the case may be. I am grateful to them and I abhor them; I ask why they happened, and yet I don't want to know the answer because there is no answer. I want to understand, and yet I think that living with what *is* is more important.

Very often I have been with people who described a situation where they found themselves in a darkness, an impasse, a tunnel without light, or a fog, triggered or made worse by some seemingly trivial loss or apparent inability to cope. And just as often then I have found myself saying that the awareness of this morass is important; that I cannot make it 'all right' by snapping them out of it; that they should not despair but 'sit' with the present situation and become more aware of it, not wish it away. All I could do was offer them my fellow-feelings – my empathy in the sense of 'feeling-in' and my companionship in the sense of being the one who shares bread (companion = with bread) with them. Someone who shares is someone who does not judge, who accepts, who is there; but this is also someone who hopes, believes and trusts: in the person, in the process and in life itself, to change and to renew. And in this change and renewal some sort of meaning is discovered.

It is this discovery of meaning which I believe to be at the heart of loss and bereavement. We live in an age when the search for meaning is becoming more and more difficult because we have instant access to gratification. The search for meaning is therefore that much harder and elusive, but also that much more important and satisfying.

By having been given the opportunity to write this book I have also been given an opportunity to discover some meaning in my losses. Perhaps, dear reader, you will spot some of my losses in these pages; perhaps you will be right and perhaps not. That is not the point. The point is that you may also be able to consider some of your own meaning by reading about mine, and thus the cycle of human achievement has advanced by a turn.

Verena Tschudin

Introduction

....

When a book is attempting to do two distinct tasks, there is a problem: which one has priority?

This book is attempting to be a text both about *counselling* and *loss and bereavement*. The idea is that those who have experienced loss and bereavement can and should be helped by counselling and counselling skills. This necessitates explaining side by side the various aspects of loss and the various skills and processes of counselling.

The Four Questions Model will be considered first, in Chapters 2–5, as a framework for counselling and helping:

What is happening?
What is the meaning of it?
What is your goal?
How are you going to do it?

This is a model which I have developed over the years and have invariably found helpful. It is by no means exclusive, and I shall make reference to other models as well. But this model can be used in various ways and by trained and untrained people.

The 'Core Conditions' as described by many of the counselling theorists:

Congruence
Warmth
Non-judgemental attitude

will be addressed particularly in Chapters 6–8, though they will also be referred to in other chapters.

Specific *counselling skills* will be addressed in Chapters 9–12:

Listening
Reflecting
Goal setting
Challenging

There are many other possible skills which will also be considered in the course of this book, but they are on the whole variations and extensions of this category of skills.

The *counselling relationship* will be considered particularly in Chapters 13 and 14:

Beginning relationships
Sustaining relationships
Ending relationships

Understanding these is vital if any real help is to be given. Knowing about relationships has to be there at the beginning when first meeting a person, but in order
to go into more detail this aspect will be dealt with specifically in Chapters 13
and 14.

Each chapter follows a similar pattern:

First, a story of the relevant topic is told.
Then follows some theoretical background and discussion of literature on the topic
    of the chapter.
Next, the counselling aspect highlighted for the particular chapter is considered.
A final putting together and synthesis follows.

This pattern is there for simplicity of writing and (hopefully) understanding; in
real life there is no such division. It may therefore be useful for the reader to dip
in and out of chapters, i.e. when reading Chapter 3 (What is the meaning of it?)
also to read some aspects of Chapter 10 (Reflecting), Chapter 8 (Empathy) and
Chapter 14 (Ending relationships). Only in this way can counselling be understood
holistically. Reading about a different aspect of loss in each chapter in this way
may also help that topic to be seen more holistically.

There are many excellent books about bereavement on the market (I was surprised that more of them were written in the 1980s than the 1990s). Some are
listed at the end of the chapters as further reading. Some of the most poignant
books are written by the bereaved themselves. Indeed, an editor once told me that
she had to reject many unsolicited manuscripts, a good number of which were
accounts of death, dying and bereavement. Perhaps these events leave such an
impression that people have to express it in book form? Perhaps all of us need to
write a book some time about our lives, even if it is never published?

Only certain aspects of loss are addressed in this book, and most of the losses
considered are not about bereavement following the loss of another person. But
all the losses described involve people and relationships. When considering the
loss of health, values or self-respect, this involves ourselves first of all, and the
relationship we have with ourselves in particular, therefore asking for self-reflec-
tionand awareness.

That only certain losses are discussed in this book is due to limitation of space
in particular, but also to limitation of experience and knowledge. While all of us
can imagine what other people are feeling and going through, our own experience
is inevitably limited. But our empathy is not limited. With empathy we can go
further than with comparison. We can also be more effective with empathy than
with sympathy (Tschudin, 1995, p. 77). Empathy makes up for what we lack in
experience, and this shows the true helping ability. But we do also need imagination: we can imagine what other situations may be experienced as loss, and therefore there is no need to be too detailed here. Since this is not a 'how-to' book –
but a book to stimulate the imagination and helping capacity – it is perhaps right

that only a certain number of situations are described. The loss of this possibility to describe is a certain gain – I hope – for the possibility to be creative in helping relationships.

The book is not written for a specific group of people or for specific study; rather it is written for all kinds of health care workers who come in contact with patients, clients, and colleagues. Among these professionals will be some who may not be very familiar with bereavement and others who are. It is perhaps the unexpected connections with loss and grief which may suddenly surface and leave one baffled. The book is mostly for people who would like to feel more comfortable with helping others to make connections, see links, and understand some aspect of life better.

As such, the book is not intended for any specific course of study either. It is not a specifically academic book, but it is not un-academic. This is deliberate, in the hope that the style and content may be applicable to many people and many fields of learning and study.

Various terms are used for the experience of loss. In popular language, loss, bereavement and grief are often used interchangeably. This may sometimes be useful, sometimes confusing. Where possible, a distinction has been made in this book between the terms, using the most appropriate word for clarity. It is not always the word itself which matters, though, but the meaning which a person gives to it, and this may have to be heard and acknowledged first.

CHAPTER ONE

Experiences of loss and bereavement

....

Everybody is an expert at loss and bereavement. This is what living is all about. It is just that not everybody is an expert at coping with loss and bereavement, or coping well with them. There are times when all of us need help with a loss, and we may need expert help at these times.

In nearly 20 years of counselling practice I have come to the conclusion that most of life's problems are caused by our experiences of loss and how we cope – or don't – with them. Loss is the cause of the problems; what is manifested, experienced and felt is that we have difficulties with relationships.

Experiences of loss

Losses of various kinds destroy, hurt, damage and diminish not just the part of life which we share with others and relate to others. They also do the same to the soul, the psyche or inner life of a person which is not as readily shared and visible. Many people are very unfamiliar with this inner life of themselves and therefore hardly recognize what is going on there. Others are aware of something but cannot access it easily. Yet others live entirely in this inner life and find it very difficult – even impossible – to relate to the outer, everyday life. These might be the people who would be described as mentally ill. Most of us are somewhere in between some of these extremes, not quite fitting any description neatly. We have also learned to adapt and change as necessary and therefore can relate to one thing one day, and something else on another day. This may be part of the puzzle of our selves and of the means we have devised to deal with loss.

Losing something does not start only with the awareness of it. In my counselling practice I have often been struck with the stories I hear clients telling me of losses very early on in their lives.

Clive, a man well into his thirties, was in his second career. He was not coping well with his work as this had also necessitated moving to a different part of the country. He had recently left his family and was in the process of divorcing. All these events were significant losses and he experienced them as such. But he only started to make sense of them and relate them to his present situation when he began to see the losses in his early life. One event stood out: when his brother was born and he effectively 'lost' his mother. This caused such problems then that he stopped eating and was force-fed by his parents. He came to see this as a loss of his identity and independence.

Clearly, Clive could not have expressed these feelings and emotions in such words, but the *fact* was still there, and this stayed with him. He realized that many of his ways of behaving and interacting with people were in fact left-overs of defence mechanisms learned when he was two or three years old but which now interfered with his life in significant ways.

Loss is an unavoidable and inextricable part of being human. It is even possible to say that we are born to die, and life can be summed up as consisting of a series of losses. Many nursing and medical authors have described the physical manifestations of loss, and the various stages of the process of adjustment to loss and bereavement, but for an understanding of loss itself, and the meaning of it, we have to go to literature, especially fiction and poetry, and particularly religious and spiritual writings.

Losing something or someone challenges our values and the meaning which we attach to life, to people, objects and ideas. In order to live successfully, we need to have and pursue a whole range of projects or goals. We may be aware of a great number of such projects, but we are probably also not aware, or at least not very obviously so, of many others of our projects. Losing an old glove may be annoying, but losing a filofax can be disastrous. Breaking an arm may mean losing some independence for a while, but getting old and ill may mean losing one's independence at a much more profound level.

The fact that loss is really only seen to be loss because it is not chosen, is significant. When we chose to do something or be with someone, we have a certain control over the situation. When this is absent we feel threatened. The meaning we give to life and living is questioned and attacked. A loss demands of us some kind of response, in the form of physical and mental adjustment. When we have had time to consider a possible response beforehand, we are again in control. But when this has not been present, we are challenged.

Life projects may consist of needs to be successful, to have good relationships, to be honest with people, to help others, to be healthy, etc. When we are prevented from fulfilling these projects, we are faced with the meaning of these ideas and pursuits. This means essentially that we are faced with the meaning of our lives and our own selves. We are faced with questions like 'Who am I?', 'What is life for?', 'What am I doing on this earth?', 'What have I done with my life?', 'Is there life after this?' These questions can really only be answered in relation to something greater than ourselves. We recognize that we are not the final arbiters of our lives when we are faced with loss, and to make sense of loss we need to participate in something which goes beyond ourselves and which is greater than our lives. It is this which is addressed when we are challenged by loss.

Loss and death attack what we are and have been and question what we will be. Life is the totality of our projects, and living successfully means linking all the projects together. When one project is lost or forced out of its position, the other projects are necessarily affected and the life pattern is distorted. Some losses can be restored, but death is final, and therefore destroys finally. This, no doubt, is why death is experienced as the final loss.

Children experience losses just as strongly as adults, but having not sufficient language to express themselves, nor the longer life experience, they react to losses on an emotional or physical level only. Clive, in the story above, was being pushed aside by his younger brother and therefore internalized this as being less important than his brother. In order to attract the attention of his parents he did the only thing which he, as a two or three year old could muster: he stopped eating. Because he could not reason, he did not see that this was in fact self-destructive at a deeper level. At a time when he should have been growing in independence and self-identity, having to be force-fed by his parents actually reduced his independence and identity. He became withdrawn. The recurring night-dreams of his childhood always ended with him falling into a deep hole at the end of the road.

Such images and experiences lead to children growing up with their personalities severely damaged. But they are not aware of this, and neither perhaps are their parents and peers. The relating they are capable of is however distorted, perhaps always marked by withdrawal, violence of one kind or another, or some form of domination. It may only be much later in life that such patterns become really problematic.

Much of our present behaviour is based on memories which may go very far back. In a moment of challenge we react physically, sometimes by being rooted to the spot, or running away or towards, needing to go to the toilet, or feeling the knees go like jelly. These reactions are expressions of deep feelings of fear, anger, humiliation or impotence. Such feelings stem from memories.

Memories are incredibly powerful. With the conscious mind we may long have forgotten something, but somewhere within, the body has not forgotten some event. Like sleeping lions suddenly woken up, memories can leap into life and overtake us with their ferocity. Memories may be triggered by all kinds of other events or thoughts. The mind makes associations and what may not be obviously linked may nevertheless be emotionally and psychically linked. It may not at first be obvious that an event or expression stirs a particular memory. Clive had become aware of a need to be true to himself, but what this meant took a long time to become clear. And even once it had been linked to his need for personal identity and self-importance, the journey to put this into practice followed a very long and often painful path.

Clearly, not all losses are that traumatic or long-lasting. Losses which happen in later life can be more easily dealt with because different mechanisms for dealing with loss have been learned, and reason and experience have also developed with physical and emotional growth.

Clearly also, not all loss needs the kind of counselling and long-term therapeutic work which Clive needed. But what does tend to happen is that when a loss is experienced, all the other significant losses which went before also make themselves felt. A person in hospital or being treated for sickness or disease may therefore be much more in touch with other losses which happened in the past. If these were not dealt with well when they happened, or have not been integrated sufficiently, then the combination of the present suffering and the past accumulated hurts may be like a powerful explosive which the least spark can ignite. This can then lead to the emotional explosions of anger, violence or outbursts so often experienced; or to doubts, loss of energy, self-respect and confidence, and possibly to self-harm and withdrawal. Any variation on the extremes are likely, as are swings from one extreme to the other.

While many people – helpers in particular – are often very

aware of traumas of present suffering, they may be oblivious
of the fact that it may be past experiences which may be
influencing a person even more than the present. Doctors and
nurses ask all their patients and clients about their past history, but they do this in order to gain a 'medical' history; they
do not, on the whole, ask for a history of emotions or psychological and spiritual appreciations of historical events. If they
did, they might be given a dusty answer: this is not their
'department'. In a psychiatric unit or hospital this would be
different. This only shows the compartmentalization which
we have introduced into our lives.

Dealing with loss

Holistic care has made great strides in nursing, but even that
can be taken to mean that a patient is 'written up' for the
services of social workers, dietitians, chaplains and specialists
of this and that service, rather than one person listening and
hearing the patient relate and voice needs and search for
possibilities. Not that the various services and experts are not
needed; they are, but not indiscriminately and not on our
judgement only.

Perhaps loss is still largely understood in terms of bereavement and the loss of a person. Very often I find myself telling
people who describe some disaster which happened, that they
are experiencing a bereavement. This is often accepted first
with incredulity and then with relief. The feelings and
emotions which they are aware of seem strangely strong and
perhaps quite unknown and unnerving. They do not recognize them as the feelings and emotions of grief. But when
this is pointed out to them they can recognize what is happening and can make sense of the situation. This is often
enough of a 'key' for people to understand what is happening
and deal with it. Sometimes it needs a little more explanation
and help to understand the context and the content. This is
when either counselling or the use of counselling skills may
be appropriate. The difference between these types of helping will be explained below.

A great deal has been written about bereavement and how
to help and cope with it. Strategies of various kinds have been
devised, and books have been written in great quantities to
help those with specific needs, and their helpers, to understand what is happening. Such books can be invaluable, or
they can be a complete 'turn-off'. People are bereaved in individual ways, and books may be following a strategy or process
model which may be quite unsuitable for someone. I know

from personal experience how I was shocked at my reactions and physical experiences. I had taught and helped many patients and families about bereavement, but when I was there myself, I had to tell myself on many occasions, 'this is grief – my grief, and my own way of experiencing it'. I had not realized how physically painful it could be. My stomach hurt, as if I had been kicked. And of course I had been. My arms just fell to my sides, useless, because there was no-one to hug. I seemed to have an endless store of tears, but they always came at the wrong moment, because the right moment for tears had been removed. People gave me books to read, out of the kindness of their hearts, but just to think that I should read about bereavement made me cross; I didn't need to *read about* it: it was all too physically real and I had difficulty dealing with that physicality, let alone with any thoughts and intellectual understanding. It was not until many months later that I dared to read. The person who helped me most had sensed the physical pain and talked about it with me. I have never forgotten her or her words and the help they represented at the time.

The help which nurses and health care personnel generally can give is mostly in allowing patients and clients to talk. Many of us are in the position of the man who said 'How do I know what I think until I have said it?'; that is, we 'discover' who and what we are in talking and expressing ourselves. Many bereaved people have an intense need to talk. Every time the story is told some aspect of it changes slightly. In this way the person changes and adapts. But this may take a long time. The gifts of time, of listening and of not being afraid to share experiences of loss, death and failure are perhaps the most precious gifts we can give one another. These commodities are often 'rationed' for many good and not so good reasons. Perhaps when using counselling and counselling skills we are also making a statement: that people are important, and by listening to them we do not only help them to understand themselves and live more satisfyingly. Sharing is one of the fundamentals of life. By listening and helping others we are helped ourselves, and by extension that means health care generally is made more humane.

Counselling and counselling skills

The word 'counselling' is used for many activities today for which it was not intended and should not be used. Etymologically it means 'giving advice', and this is the use to which the word is often put. But this is precisely what is *not* intended.

Giving advice is necessary in teaching or educational settings, but not when helping with emotional problems. In that setting the person usually needs someone who is non-judgemental, warm and congruent. When these elements are present, the person can begin a process of self-awareness leading to insight and the discovery of meaning, eventually producing goals for change.

It is usually believed that such a process of change needs help from someone independent and trained in the skills of helping. What these skills are has been extensively researched and described. As this book is not intended to be a basic text on counselling, some works are listed at the end of this chapter where readers can gain more information. However, throughout this text there will be indications for dealing with situations of loss and bereavement in a counselling framework.

The difference between 'counselling' and 'counselling skills' has been described clearly by the British Association for Counselling (BAC) in its *Code of Ethics and Practice for Counsellors* (BAC, 1993) and its *Code of Ethics and Practice for Counselling Skills* (BAC, 1989). Simply put, the significant difference is a contract. Many people use counselling skills regularly as part of their helping. These skills consist primarily of means of attending, through listening, staying open and encouraging; and challenging, through confronting with reality, self-sharing and empowering. Only when these skills are used in a regular way for helping a person, and both the client and helper agree to this help is counselling taking place.

A contract in such a counselling and helping situation can be a few words of agreement or a written document. The form of the agreement is not as significant as the fact of the agreement. A contract may also be for just one session or for a specific number of sessions. When a contract exists, 'the overall aim of counselling is to provide an opportunity for the client to work towards living in a more satisfying and resourceful way' (BAC, 1993). Both parties have to agree to this. It should be stressed that such a contract only applies to this aspect of any help given.

People who use the title of counsellor use counselling skills, but people who use counselling skills are not necessarily counsellors. Using counselling skills as part of work is very commendable and more and more expected in the health care professions. If such people also use contracts with clients, then clearly they have to be confident that they have not only the necessary counselling skills, but also the skills of forming, sustaining and ending helping relationships which might be necessary in any work they may be doing. This normally takes some considerable training, undertaken with supervision.

Anyone who calls herself or himself a counsellor should at least abide by the Code of Ethics of the BAC, even though it is not necessary to belong to the BAC. This Code enjoins on counsellors to have regular supervision of case work. This is not only good practice, but is also a safeguard for clients. To undertake work as a counsellor is not done lightly, but neither should it not be undertaken because of lack of confidence; this is precisely where supervision is invaluable. And what we help others to do, we should have experienced ourselves at least to some degree: if we try to empower others, we should have been empowered ourselves. Having supervision is not just a bonus, but something vital and professionally required. People who use counselling skills are not required to have supervision for their work in the same way, but it is nevertheless highly recommended even here.

Culture and religion

The culture, mores and traditions of individuals and societies are particularly important in the area of death, dying and bereavement. It has been said that a people can be judged by the kind of cemeteries it keeps. If this is true, then our British cemeteries are on the whole indeed a reflection of the place we afford to bereavement: small, neat, clean and no-fuss. Many people find the emphasis on dying in eastern religions and cultures strange and even morbid. 'The day of death is more important than the day of birth' (Dalai Lama, 1995) is the reverse of what the West has come to accept.

If the expectation is that death should be 'sanitized' as much as possible, then the experience of many people is just the opposite. The more the physical signs of a death and bereavement have to be controlled or made to disappear, the more the psyche may compensate and suffer. The emotions and feelings may then take on a life of their own, growing in importance and refusing to remain silent. Perhaps it is not surprising that we are therefore a materialist society, needing many possessions to give security to our lives because we have lost the security which the connection with life beyond the grave had previously given.

Health care workers are in a unique position to help people who may be suffering because of locked-up feelings and emotions – 'unfinished business' – concerning loss and grief in their clients and patients. It is often in quite unrelated moments that such needs come to light. Not only suppressed feelings may need to be responded to, but in people of different cultures, specific rituals or beliefs may need to be respected which may be carried on or held while in contact with health professionals.

Counselling is not a form of help which is imposed, but is at best offered tentatively. Where a need arises for help, counselling skills are never out of place, because the skills of listening and reflecting are universally welcome. What should be respected though is that if a need is discovered, and the client or patient refuses help – because the custom may be that the family should help – this must be acknowledged, even if it means watching a situation being handled differently from what may be 'simple' or 'obvious'. This is not always easy, and may even tax a helper's skills and personal worth. This applies to the subject of this book only – not of course to situations where other interventions are called for.

Further reading

Suggested further reading on counselling theories and skills

Burnard, P. (1992) *Counselling: A Guide to Practice in Nursing*. Oxford: Butterworth-Heinemann.

Burnard, P. (1994) *Counselling Skills for Health Professionals* (2nd edn). London: Chapman & Hall.

Egan, G. (1994) *The Skilled Helper* (5th edn). Belmont, CA: Brooks/Cole Publishing.

Howe, D. (1993) *On Being a Client: Understanding the Process of Counselling*. London: Sage.

Nelson-Jones, R. (1993) *Practical Counselling and Helping Skills* (3rd edn). London: Cassell.

Nelson-Jones, R. (1993) *Training Manual for Counselling and Helping Skills*. London: Cassell.

Tschudin, V. (1994) *Counselling; A Primer for Nurses. Workbook and Workshop Guide*. London: Baillière Tindall.

Tschudin, V. (1995) *Counselling Skills for Nurses* (4th edn). London: Baillière Tindall.

Suggested further reading for religion and culture

Kalisch, R.A. (1977) *Death and Dying: Views from Many Cultures*. New York: Baywood.

Penson, J. (1990) *Bereavement: A Guide for Nurses*. London: Harper and Row.

Rinpoche, S. (1992) *The Tibetan Book of Living and Dying*. London: Rider.

CHAPTER TWO

Loss of a life partner
What is happening?

Harry had been a very successful financial dealer in the City. He and his wife Rosalyn had a close and loving marriage. They had three children, two boys aged 14 and 12 and a little girl of six. Three years ago Harry, now 42 and with a comfortable life-style, had decided that he would prefer to spend the rest of his life teaching. Rosalyn supported him all the way, and he went to Cambridge to read literature. The family went with him there for the two years of his course. On finishing, they had a great party to which they had invited many friends at their family home. The morning after the party Rosalyn found Harry dead beside her when she woke up; he had died of a heart attack in the night.

Rosalyn was now in hospital, six months after that event, with a badly fractured right ankle, sustained while tripping on an uneven pavement.

Jane was 60 when she was diagnosed to have carcinoma of the ovary which had already metastasized. Her husband, Donald, and she had married only 15 years earlier; they had no children. Jane only had an elderly cousin in another part of the country, and Donald had no family other than his elderly parents. Jane had received all the usual treatments, but despite this the disease had progressed rapidly. They were both active church goers and many in their congregation had supported Jane and Donald with concern and prayer, also helping Jane with housework and shopping. Jane was very much aware of her prognosis and she and Donald had always shared news, feelings, hopes and fears. Jane was convinced that the prayerful concern of their many friends had helped her to stay in control and only when she had become too uncomfortable and it was clear that she was dying, was the decision taken to give her an injection of morphine. Jane even thanked the nurse and, holding Donald's hand, died a few minutes later.

Later in the same year Donald's parents also died, within weeks of each other.

Nearly two years after this, Donald discovered that he had cancer of the prostate. He was admitted to hospital where he was operated on and later had a course of radiotherapy.

These two stories of bereavements could not be more dissimilar. In the first story, the significant element is the suddenness, the shock and the total disbelief which Rosalyn experienced, and which marked her bereavement. After the funeral the two boys declared that they could never again believe in a God, whatever anybody might say. Rosalyn experienced this as an added burden.

Donald, on the other hand, had done most of his grieving with Jane, and after her death there was mostly relief. The fact that his parents died in the same year meant that the actual process of grieving for his wife was interrupted and had to be re-focused twice over. This was not easy, and has perhaps been the element which has left the bigger mark on his psyche. Finding that he had cancer also needed a great deal of new adjustment and facing of fears.

The death of a spouse

In their famous 'social readjustment scale' Holmes and Rahe (1967, in Penson, 1990, p. 14) rate the death of a spouse as 100 units. The next closest event is listed as divorce, worth 73 units. Between 60 and 80 units is considered an average amount of stress, but above 100 there is risk of serious ill-effect. Donald's score might be:

100	death of a spouse
126	death of close family member (63 each)
53	major personal injury or illness
279	

This is a dangerous score, though it would depend on Donald's personality and ways of coping, and also on the time interval between events. The closer together they happen, the longer the score will remain high.

The following elements are common to most aspects of loss and bereavement. As they have been particularly developed in the arena of the death of a spouse, they are detailed here, but will be referred to also in later parts of the book.

The grieving process

It was Colin Murray Parkes who, in the 1960s and 1970s, brought bereavement into the open with several publications stemming from his research with London widows (e.g. Parkes, 1964; 1970; 1971; 1975a). Parkes was concerned to classify grief in terms of medical diagnosis, and for this reason he tried to understand the components of grief and see this as a process. He listed three stages of grieving (Parkes, 1975a, p. 21):

numbness
pining
depression

and says that only after the stage of depression can recovery occur.

Kübler-Ross (1969) has described five stages of grieving when dying. These stages have also been applied to people who grieve after the death of a loved one:

Denial
Anger
Bargaining
Depression
Acceptance.

Speck (1978, pp. 10–12) describes three aspects of grief work, which he calls:

Shock and disbelief
Developing awareness
Resolution.

Worden (1991, p. 10) divides mourning into four tasks, rather than stages:

To accept the reality of the loss
To work through to the pain of grief
To adjust to an environment in which the deceased is missing
To emotionally relocate the deceased and move on with life.

These stages have become so well known that it is difficult to think in other ways about grieving and helping the bereaved. It is perhaps significant that Parkes (1975a) wrote about 'stages' with reference to a medical model of disease. Speck (1978, p. 13) says that these stages are 'general framework(s) ... to describe how people may reassess their world, and themselves in relation to it, following the experience of a major personal loss'. When thinking in holistic terms, it may however be useful to suspend the idea of stages altogether. All the authors make the point that people do not necessarily pass through the stages smoothly; indeed they may go through all the stages in the space of a few minutes

(Tschudin, 1995, p. 119), again and again. Helping of whatever kind means essentially being with the person where she or he is at the moment – in or out of a framework – working with the possibility that there may be many other factors which may be present, and perhaps more important at this moment than anything stated. Stages, frameworks and models have their place, giving helpers the possibility to work more effectively by not having to start at the beginning each time. But all such theory needs also to be dispensable in the effort to be human and to address the person rather than the problem. Grieving is a natural response to loss and applying a 'medical model' may therefore give a wrong impression. It is even difficult to say when the natural response becomes 'unnatural', that is, when grieving becomes pathological. All the models will be referred to and used in this book at relevant points.

Commitment

Both Parkes (1975a) and Bowlby (1980) make the point strongly that grieving only takes place because we are 'attached' to people, and committed to them. We cannot in the same way mourn some stranger far away as we mourn the person with whom we shared life for many years. The commitment brings joy and security, satisfaction, growth and comfort. But the cost of the commitment is great when all these things are destroyed with the death of the one who 'personified' them. Nevertheless, most people would prefer to make the commitment rather than remain uncommitted for fear of the possible pain on losing the person. People who do not marry or live in a one-to-one partnership still normally commit themselves to causes or ideas, and the 'significant others' are widely recognized as valid descriptions of relationships.

The commitment to the loved person is often seen most clearly if the person is suffering or slowly dying. Despite the fact that some people say that she or he is no longer the person they married, or that they feel the dying person is no longer a 'person', they would find it difficult not to care for that person. This time of caring and leave-taking is often of the greatest importance. The anticipatory grief work allows for absorbing the reality of the loss gradually; finishing any unfinished business and possibly resolving past conflicts; beginning to change assumptions about life and the identity of those concerned; and making plans for the future which may then not be considered as betrayals of the deceased after death (Rando, 1984, p. 37). Gass and Chang (1989) found that '(t)he opportunity for anticipatory grieving was one resource which likely contributed to [the widowed persons'] resource strength', helping them to manage before and after bereavement.

Normal grieving

The circumstances of the death of the spouse matter more than anything in the grieving which has to be done. Young or old, a quick death or a slow one, a 'good' death or a 'bad' one – and endless variations in between – matter enormously how the remaining spouse will cope.

Many people find the death of someone a relief. This perhaps indicates that much anticipatory grieving has been done.

On the other hand, when someone dies unexpectedly, the shock can be so great that it can literally paralyse a person.

Normal grieving is therefore a very flexible concept and must always be seen in relation to the whole person and how she or he behaved before the death of the spouse.

The stage of shock and denial

This first phase after the death of a spouse is invariably marked by shock and a certain numbness (Parkes, 1970): 'I can't take it all in'; 'I can't believe it'. Even when a death has been anticipated, it is difficult to imagine beforehand how the world will be without the loved one, and when the person has died, it is difficult to take in that the body, still exactly the same form, is now not alive.

Those people whose spouses die in accidents, or where there may be no body, as in major disasters, inevitably have more difficulty with the first reaction to death. While the knowledge may always be there that one day we die, in the course of daily living this is not what most people occupy their thoughts with. It is not surprising that the first reaction to the death is therefore 'No, it can't be'.

This time of numbness is usually relatively short, lasting from some hours to some days. Parkes (1970) points out, however, that some form of denial is quite common even a year after the death.

The stage of developing awareness

When the initial numbness has passed, the feelings, which may have been held back, come to the fore, and a time of chaos and swings in all directions begins. Kübler-Ross (1969) speaks of anger, bargaining and depression, and Bowlby and Parkes (1970) speak of disorganization, yearning and protest. Parkes (1970) describes protest as a 'restless irritability or bitterness toward others or the self'; and yearning as pangs of intense longing or pining to reunite with the lost object.

Anger tends to be directed at the deceased for having died, leaving the spouse or family, but also against those who might have helped, such as members of the family, doctors, nurses or emergency services. Anger at God, or fate, for allowing something so terrible to happen, is very common. When anger is turned towards the self it becomes guilt. Such feelings often concern trivial things: Parkes (1970) cites a widow feeling guilt for not having made her husband a bread pudding; a client revealed her guilt for having refused her husband's request to listen to a particular record which she disliked.

In a time of surging feelings and disorganization, the pendulum swings from denial to acceptance and back again. But all the time the swings become less extreme and an awareness grows from which the person can view life again with some equanimity. It should not be forgotten, though, that 'an abnormal reaction to an abnormal situation is normal' (Frankl, 1962, p.18). While bereavement is common, it is nevertheless an 'abnormal' situation for each person concerned.

The stage of resolution

After a time of disorganization, a reorganization will eventually emerge. This is not a going back to life as it was, but there is an acceptance of a new state of affairs. The spouse has found a new identity as widow or widower, there is a detachment from the deceased which is healthy. The widowed person can talk again about the spouse without crying and with realism, able to acknowledge good and bad times, good and bad characteristics in the deceased.

Families and friends often await this stage eagerly in the widowed person. They themselves may have reached this stage much earlier than the spouse and they may be impatient with her or him for still being 'stuck' somewhere in the past. It is impossible to be precise when someone should have come 'through' a bereavement and function again normally. As a very general rule it is possible to say that about two years from the death is reasonable for normal grief to resolve. But some times may be harder to cope with, such as anniversaries, and there may be some aspects of grieving which will always be present, although the person can be said to have accepted the new reality.

Many people say that they can forgive but not forget, and this is entirely reasonable. Remembering is a very important function of living: we are what we are through an accumulation of events and participation in them, and we cannot divorce their memories from us. Not all of the memories are good, and what disturbs people are the bad or painful memories. Remembering the bad or painful things will not change them. We can choose, however, *how* we remember them, that is, what we do with the memories: we can let them hurt us or we can accept them simply as memories. This is perhaps the distinction between a grieving process which is prolonged and therefore becomes pathological, and a process which is resolved.

Helping the bereaved person

Counselling is essentially a form of help which prompts and then draws on the client's own resources and strengths. But someone who is newly bereaved cannot be not in touch with those resources and strengths. Someone in the stage of shock and denial needs practical help to cope with daily activities. This may involve much direct giving of instruction: 'do this now'; 'go there for that'. The helping to be done at this moment is essentially of being close as a person, doing tasks as necessary, supporting and accepting.

When a bereaved person is beginning to move towards the stage of developing awareness, then counselling skills become useful. This stage is characterized by emotions, feelings, mood swings, experiences of deep pain and confusion. This time demands sensitive listening, a non-judgemental attitude and an understanding that a helper is there with and for the bereaved in a very direct and congruent way.

In this stage the person often needs to talk a great deal. The 'story' of the death and surrounding events has to be repeated again and again. Everybody who comes in contact with the bereaved person is told. Those who help the bereaved may have to listen to the same story many times. The value in listening is that the helper will hear how the story changes and moves on. If this does not happen, this may be an indication that more concrete help needs to be given.

Telling the story over and over is therapeutic for the bereaved person. While the bereaved was in a state of shock and denial the event seems to have happened 'out there'; the denial is a form of protection against being hurt by something awful. People describe this time as one of 'cotton wool' (Speck, 1978, p. 11) or like being wrapped in an invisible blanket (Lewis, 1961, p. 7), or like being numb and solid (Parkes, 1970). In such a state it is almost impossible to take anything in, and the event seems to be happening in a film that is being watched. By telling the story gradually the 'film' becomes reality; it no longer happens 'out there' but becomes 'in here'. Hence the confusion and the feelings which are all over the place. To find some order in their situation, the person has to talk and hear herself or himself say the impossible, painful or outrageous.

Those who help people at that time can do this best by using counselling skills: listening, reflecting and gently challenging so that the story can change and movement can happen.

It is only when this phase becomes well established that counselling as such – with a contract, however tentative, between helper and bereaved person – can begin. So that the disparate and often unexpected and painful feelings which mark this time can be examined, understood and used to effect, many people find it helpful to talk with someone experienced in both counselling and bereavement. Neither is necessary, as long as the helper is aware of her or his limits and is able to take appropriate steps.

What is happening?

When it is clear that the help to be given is because of a bereavement, this question is a very good way in to helping. 'Tell me what happened' is a way of giving permission to talk, perhaps at length.

Helping another person by using counselling skills is gentle, not imposing, and is there entirely for the client or patient, that is, the nurse is not looking for information to use in putting together a care plan.

The fact that a question is asked is an opening, an invitation; it is not a command. It is easy enough for a person to answer in such a way that it is understood if the person does not want to talk.

But the question 'what is happening?' is essential for several reasons and purposes:

to give permission to talk
to invite to talk
to convey 'you are OK'
      'I am here to listen'
      'I am here just for you'
      'I want to hear what you have to say'
      'I am not shocked'
      'I care about you'
      'It matters to me what you have to say'.

When we ask this question we must necessarily be willing to hear the answer, and it may be a long answer. It is positively harmful to invite someone to talk and after a few minutes give the impression that we are not interested any more. If there is no time it may be better not to invite someone to talk. It may then be more honest to say that there is no time, but give an indication when there might be time. This would constitute a contract and may be very helpful.

Body language and symptoms of physical pain can be important indicators for health care workers to notice and be aware of. There is plenty of anecdotal evidence of people being admitted to hospital with severe attacks of arthritis every year about the same time; of showing the same symptoms of disease as those which a spouse died of; of people interpreting pain and disease as consequences of events or bad actions. There is no official medical diagnosis of a 'broken heart', but Parkes (1975a, p. 29) quotes a source from the year 1657, detailing causes of death in London, in which ten cases were attributed to grief. Claims have been made that cancer can follow bereavement but it would be hard to prove this scientifically. In the mind of a person it may not be such a hard conclusion to reach.

It can be helpful to consider physical pain as manifestations of emotional states:

Pain in the chest can be indicative of 'heart-ache' and pining for a dead person.

Pain in the abdomen can say 'I have been kicked in the stomach'.

Pain in the throat can point to being left speechless in the face of a death. It could also point to a need or desire to give a 'mouthful' to someone, but not daring.

Aching arms may point to their redundancy now that the loved person cannot be hugged or cuddled any more.

Pain on swallowing can reflect that the person cannot or could not swallow what happened.

Nausea may be a manifestation of feeling sick at the sight of funerals, or any other particular memory with the dead person.

An aware helper may be able to interpret many signs and symptoms in similar and sensitive ways. It is never the case that something *is* like that, but *may be* or *may point to* some way of seeing and understanding a situation.

What is happening to Rosalyn?

Rosalyn was in hospital with a broken ankle. Presumably on her admission she told the nurses that she was widowed, and it is likely that a few words were exchanged between Rosalyn and the nurse on this topic, but the reason for her admission was the fracture, not the bereavement.

The 'broken' ankle may make a connection to Rosalyn's 'broken' heart. When asking a person 'what is happening?' it may be helpful to offer such connections and in this way help them to see links between the body and the emotions or the body and the soul, the visible and the invisible. Being able to concentrate for a few moments on the word 'broken' may bring to mind many other memories which may suddenly have been refreshed, sometimes for no apparent reasons.

It must be stressed though that these are suggestions, not rules, and not everybody may find this helpful. The cue should always be taken from the person herself or himself as to how much they might be in touch with their own feelings and understanding.

A bereavement is, on the whole, a physically painful experience. The body has received a shock, especially when the person died suddenly, as was the case for Rosalyn. The person often referred to 'my better half' has been torn away violently – even if the death was not violent. There was no preparation for such a parting. The fact that the other person represented the 'better half' of oneself shows how much projection often takes place, of the good personal attributes we would like to have but somehow never manage to acquire, or which, for one reason or another, we are quite happy to project on to the other person. This means essentially that we do not consider ourselves either as good as the other person, or we idolize the other. In any case, it means that we do not feel as competent, fulfilled, self-sufficient or whole. When therefore the person, who represented all these wishes or dreams, dies without notice, it is possible to feel angry for:

not making provision for a 'better' life
not helping the spouse to gain confidence
taking the 'better' part into the grave
being left stranded emotionally and materially.

It is possible that Rosalyn felt these and similar things. Unable perhaps, to cope with them, she may have needed a space where she could be helped, and her subconscious may have 'arranged' a 'break' and a possibility to get help legitimately.

Even if this may have been picked up by a health care professional, Rosalyn may not yet have been able to express her needs freely. It may therefore be that she may be crying a great deal, or be withdrawn, or refuse to eat. In other words, she may exhibit some behaviour to draw attention to herself. Once she has attention, she may still not be articulate enough to say 'I need help'. It is therefore important for those who help others to be open. The question 'what is happening?' is particularly helpful. But with their emphasis on action and 'making things right' nurses are always in danger of focusing on the practical, obvious and clearly health or illness related aspects. This question asks also for the emotional, psychological, not-so-obvious, intangible and perhaps hidden part of the person.

Neither the practical and obvious, nor the emotional and spiritual, should be ignored. Holistic care means that all aspects of a person are given the attention needed. This may change from day to day. When we are willing to help someone with counselling and counselling skills, we need to be aware particularly of the emotional side of the person. And the key to that is often a clear and unambiguous indication that we are willing to hear *that* side now.

What is happening to Donald?

If we want to help others we need to start where they start, go to where they are, acknowledge their reference points and align our reference points to theirs.

Donald and Jane had been very close right up to the moment of Jane's death. Donald will therefore have done a great deal of anticipatory grieving and the phase of shock and numbness (Chapter 1) may therefore not be very evident. He may also have learned already what it is like to go back into an empty house, however difficult that may have been before Jane died.

In the phase of developing awareness, many bereaved

people report occasions of seeing or hearing the dead person. Because this is something they are not accustomed to, they fear that they are going mad and this may therefore add to their distress.

One well-known phenomenon is the hallucinatory (usually known as psychic or religious) experience of the dead person. The bereaved person becomes aware of the dead in a very real way which is difficult to describe. But there is no doubt for the experiencer that it is real.

Soon after my husand died – I cannot say how long – a few days or even hours – I saw him crossing a plank bridge which had been thrown across a stream.

The stream was in the midst of glorious country and there were fresh green bushes and trees everywhere. The plank was old gnarled wood, not very wide and had evidently been utilized solely in order to get across the water. It was as simple as that.

His pace was slow but very sure. He never turned round, yet I felt that he was aware that I was following at a distance.

I could not see anything beyond his figure.

I had no doubt whatever that he would be lovingly received when he reached his destination (Maxwell and Tschudin, 1990, p. 93).

Such experiences are quite frequent (Baro *et al.*, 1986), but have been viewed with suspicion in the Christian tradition, equating them more with primitive cults or spiritualism. This is slowly changing as more studies about bereavement become available where such events are related. For those who have such experiences, they tend to be a comfort and also play a helpful part in the adjustment to grieving. In the experience quoted, the narrator was obviously reassured about her husband's fate: he would be lovingly received on the other side of the water dividing her world from his. This is not only a reassurance, but a realization that the dead person is in fact now in an other dimension and *is* dead.

Donald may or may not have had such an experience, and may or may not have told his nurses about it. The fact that he suffered three bereavements within the space of a few months may have made such experiences more likely. Donald would probably have described himself as a down-to-earth type of person and not given much to extrasensory perceptions. The fact that such hallucinations can happen to anyone may have taken him very much by surprise and may have worried him.

In counselling and helping it may be possible to ask, 'have

you ever had an experience of Jane after her death?' and this may trigger a memory. This is not just an idle question or inquisitiveness. Many people are genuinely helped by such experiences, and given permission, bereaved people may be enabled to allow themselves to venture into unknown territory. The question 'what is happening?' is not restricted to those particular words. It is a very general question which covers many aspects of asking for more information, more putting together of events, memories and feelings. The question can and should be asked of as many people as possible who are involved in a situation. The more that a situation can be seen to relate to all of life, the more the death can also be seen in the context of that life.

The fact that Donald had lost his three closest relatives in a very short time meant that he had barely had time to mourn for Jane when his mother died. Although he was not emotionally as close to her as he was to Jane, it nevertheless will have brought up other feelings and memories which will have to be addressed also. The newest loss often means that other losses become much more alive again and may have to be dealt with more urgently than the present loss. Indeed, the present loss may fade into the background, and this may puzzle helpers who may not have any connection with the earlier loss.

The loss of parents (see Chapter 3) brings quite different aspects to light which may have to be mourned, and therefore Donald may have had to deal with a considerable burden of feelings which demanded his attention. As he was in hospital two years after the death of Jane, it may be thought that he should have done his main grieving for her. Two years is considered a normal time span for the acute grieving phase. But it must not be forgotten that Donald now faced also the grieving for his health (see Chapter 7) and this with the same disease from which Jane died. His many kinds and types of grieving will therefore have made a big impact – even in someone stoical and thinking himself level-headed. This should not be overlooked. On the other hand, it should not be assumed either that because he may not give the impression of suffering, that he is denying his suffering.

'What is happening?' is a universal question. It never hurts to ask this question. The answer given will however need careful interpretation. The response made will depend on it – and that can be for better or for worse. Asking 'what is happening?' may be risky – but living is risky.

....

Further reading Lewis, C.S. (1961) *A Grief Observed*. London: Faber & Faber.

Stroebe, W. & Stroebe, M.S. (1987) *Bereavement and Health: The Psychological and Physical Consequences of Partner Loss*. Cambridge: Cambridge University Press.

Wallbank, S. (1992) *The Empty Bed: Bereavement and the Loss of Love*. London: Darton, Longman & Todd.

Znaniecka Lopata, H. (1996) *Current Widowhood; Myths and Realities*. London: Sage.

CHAPTER THREE

Loss of a parent
What is the meaning of it?

Audrey, aged 47, had always had a difficult relationship with her mother, aged 83. Both of them were very strong personalities. A series of events had led Audrey to leave a job, home, and a circle of friends. She had become destitute and might have had to be admitted to a psychiatric hospital, had her mother not made room for her in her house. Audrey moved in with her mother, and they tried to look after each other. Audrey tried her hand at some small jobs, but they never lasted. She often did not have the energy to get up in the morning, and the evenings were often spent alone in her room, with a bottle of alcohol. The relationship between mother and daughter was none too happy.

But gradually Audrey realized that her mother gave her a great deal. They managed to have the odd 'deep' conversation, as Audrey called them. One day the mother informed Audrey that she knew that something was not right with her inside, and an ultrasound scan revealed metastatic cancer. Audrey was given to understand that her mother had only a very short time to live. This was a shock to Audrey and helped her to see her mother in a new light. They talked as much as they could. Mother and daughter forgave each other for their past hurts, they enjoyed each other's company, prepared little treats for each other and seemed to re-live large parts of their lives which had been difficult, now turning them into times of joy and contentment.

Audrey's mother died very peacefully a few weeks later. The change in Audrey has lasted, and the gratitude which she felt towards her mother before her death has also been the source of energy to continue with life afterwards. She has gone back to her earlier expertise, physiotherapy, working as an assistant, part-time, in a small hospital, where her colleagues and clients value her contribution.

Beth was 13, her sister Karen was eight, and her brother Jon was 16. They lived in a mining village and their father had been a miner all his life. Four years earlier he was involved in an accident over-

ground which resulted in such injuries that he died ten days later. His wife, Susan, was devastated and never wanted to, nor could she, forgive the person whose carelessness had caused the accident. The children grew up hating this man and his family, who lived in the same village.

Susan had found it increasingly hard to cope with her responsibilities for the children. Despite a lot of help from neighbours, family and friends, she grew more and more depressed and kept to herself. Sometimes there was no food in the house and the children either went hungry or asked to go to their friends for dinner. Susan had a good pension and although money was tight, it should not have been a worry. But there was increasingly less money available for normal living. The children vacillated between wanting to care for their mother and hating her for not caring for them. They increasingly looked to their school friends for company and advice, but nobody seemed able or willing to help in a practical way. Those who showed interest were rebuffed by Susan's refusal of help.

Beth was the first back from school one day, and not seeing Susan in the house, went looking for her. After a fruitless search she began to look for her in the house. She found her finally, dead, under the duvet in her bed, with clothes heaped on top of her to make it look less obvious. She had died from an overdose of anti-depressants, washed down with a liberal helping of alcohol.

Years later Beth trained as a nurse, partly in reaction to her experience, she said, and partly in an effort to 'make good'.

No two stories of bereavement are ever likely to be the same. Bereavement is an intensely personal experience, depending very much on the relationships with the person concerned, of the expectations of the relationship, and of one's own life so far. The biggest factor here is whether one loses a parent as an adult or as a child.

Adults losing parents

In our culture it becomes increasingly rare for people actually to witness a death. This has contributed to the taboo which generally surrounds death, and therefore people who are associated with death and mourning. A man of over 50 once 'confessed' to me that he had never seen a dead body. This worried him in the sense that he thought it might help him to know what death looks like.

There is something 'normal' about someone dying in old-age. We refer to the 'three score years and ten' allotted to people in the Bible (Psalm 90: 10), and although the average life-expectancy for people in the West is slightly more than

70 years, that figure still seems an acceptable span of life. We are not surprised when an old person dies.

But ageing and old age tend to bring a decline in health and vigour and this is can cause both physical and mental suffering and anguish. In such a state many people prefer to be dead. The economic conditions also contribute to elderly people often feeling that they are in the way and would be better off dead.

This message may be passed on to children, who may themselves be adults and may be torn between caring for an elderly parent and pursuing their family life.

Matthiesen (1989) found guilt and grief to be the two most common emotions in daughters who had placed their mothers in nursing homes. These daughters expected that their feelings would only change with the death of their mothers, but this may be a questionable expectation. Raphael (1984, p. 309) suggests that younger females and the unmarried are people who need most help with a bereavement of a parent. This may indicate that these groups of people are those who may have placed their parents in nursing homes in order to carry on their life and career. The relationship between elderly parents and their often equally ageing children can be fraught with difficulty which is only partly resolved with death. Tradition and culture may then bear very heavily on such adult children after the death, expecting them to be free of 'trouble', when in fact the results of difficult relationships may only just begin to show itself. To this can be added the notion, put forward by Freud, that psychotherapy is not possible with people near or over the age of 50 (Scrutton, 1989, p. 19). This idea is certainly disputed, but nevertheless culturally still often evident.

When elderly parents die unexpectedly, many old and painful memories, which may never have been resolved, may surface. Chick (1989), in her novel poignantly entitled *I Never Told Her I Loved Her*, describes a stormy relationship with her mother. When her mother died suddenly, she found that guilt and grief (p. 68) dominated her behaviour. Wishing that others would feel rejected as she did, that others hated her as she wanted to hate them, and feeling swamped by duty (p. 72) are only some of the emotions she writes about.

When someone close dies there is almost always the sense of something unfinished. We should have said something, or done something more. At such moments we are acutely aware of our shortcomings in relationships. Some people can cope with this, but others have a need to make up for such shortcomings by keeping a room or house as the dead person had left it, or filling the house with flowers, or never laughing again. Such rituals are understandable for a while, but eventually they show that not one person has died, but two: the second one emotionally.

Part of the grieving process is to come to terms with the unfinished business, and with carrying on with life, because life carries on with us. It has often been said that we do not mourn the dead person so much as *our* loss and our own lost life. This is something which may not be well understood at first, but eventually this may have to be realized and acted on.

The scenario in Audrey's story could not be more different. As much as an unexpected death may leave unhappiness, so an unexpected reconciliation may also leave one baffled. Why could a relationship not have been sorted out earlier? This may be a legitimate question, but one which it is hard to answer reasonably. The only sure thing is that imminent and expected death concentrates the mind. Many of us will have been asked at some time, if we only had a day to live, what would we be doing? And most of us would then probably have answered that we wanted certain relationships put right. Many people find it difficult to give the gift of love in the best way possible, and it may indeed be too late one day. When, like with Audrey and her mother, the gift can be given, it is one of the greatest and most liberating gifts people can give to each other.

The grief then suffered after the death may not be typical. Indeed, some people may find themselves on a 'high' which seems puzzling to those concerned, and to those close to the bereaved person, quite unnatural. When a life has been ended well, it seems as if the energy created by that is then captured by those left behind. The sheer relief from caring for someone, which may have been relentless, may also contribute to such a feeling of elation, at least for some time. The sense of wellbeing may sometimes last for weeks, and when it does finish, it tends to be an event which may recall another relationship – this time a less good one – which causes the 'coming down to earth'.

Children losing parents

The world has always had a special care for orphans, and throughout history – and especially in literature – orphans have been the concern of interest and pity; they have also been exploited mercilessly.

In societies with welfare systems intact, orphaned children

are normally cared for adequately, at least physically. The emotional scars, however, may not appear until later in life.

Children often experience the death of a parent with a sense that it is their fault. Raphael (1984) details at great length the varying needs, behaviours and emotions of children bereaved at different ages, including adolescence. Rando (1984, p. 154) says that '(m)ost of what is true for adults in grief also holds true in age-appropriate ways for children'. When children express that it may be their fault that a parent dies, this may therefore not be too dissimilar to the adult sense of guilt. Children see and experience the world in simple black-and-white ways, whereas adults have learned to be sophisticated about their feelings and how they express these feelings.

Several authors (Oswin, 1991; Rando, 1984; Raphael, 1984), when describing the needs of bereaved children, mention their fear or anticipation of moving house. Having lost something well known, children may not like to lose other well-known objects. Just as adults become stressed when losing too many known and loved things at the same time (Penson, 1990, p. 14), so children have their own ways of expressing their needs.

That children can and do survive bereavement and grow into well-adjusted adults has been demonstrated by Simmons (1992), Cohen (1994) and Heinzer (1995).

Whether children can understand and should attend funerals has often been debated. The general consensus appears to be that they should. Penson (1990, p. 88) describes how some pupils attended the funeral of one of their friends, and the dead boy's mother, seeing his best friend there, experienced this 'like the sun breaking through the clouds, though it was still raining, [and] she stopped weeping, smiled, waved and blew him a kiss'. The fact of attending the funeral was not only important for the boy himself, but helped the bereaved parent too.

Oswin (1991), who made a study of bereavement amongst people who have learning difficulties, stresses again and again that listening to the bereaved person is vitally important. The fact that many people (not only those with special needs) may have difficulties expressing themselves does not mean that they have no feelings. Both Simmons (1992) and Cohen (1994) also stress the fact that children need to be heard and given opportunities to express themselves, both at home and in school, when they have been bereaved. Indeed, both Simmons and Cohen describe workshops and group activities for bereaved children.

The children in the scenario at the beginning of the chapter were uniquely disadvantaged. Despite much official and unofficial caring going on, it is still possible to slip through the net of agencies set up for helping. It may have been that Beth and her siblings did not want to have anybody help them and they wanted to protect their mother in her own bereavement and therefore put on a brave face whenever help might have been suggested. Their mother, too, may have clung on to them as the only treasures left after her husband's death. She may at first have found solace in looking after them and having to combine the role of both parents in herself. Despite the fact that they lived in a fairly close-knit community, nobody may really have known the state of affairs. A lone parent, bereaved herself, Susan may not have had the courage to ask for help, and in a moment of loneliness and depression, may have decided that the easiest way out of an intractable situation was suicide.

By becoming a nurse, Beth had clearly come through her bereavement in the sense that she had not only learned something, but also felt able to give something to others of her experience. This is not always the case; indeed, too many people want or need to help others out of an unmet need in themselves to be comforted.

What is the meaning of it?

The second question in the Four Questions Model tries to make sense of the given situation. Anything which we experience strongly, evokes the cry, 'why?' Why did this happen? Why now? Why to me? In order to come to terms with an event, we have to relate ourselves and our whole life to it; at least, that is what it seems to demand in terms of energy. Something either effectively trivial or experienced as trivial, does not need the same amount of emotional energy.

But the question 'why?' usually has an answer starting with 'because'. This answer looks for a reason which we can relate to and which fits our frame of reference. It is evident that we ask why a particular accident happened, and the answer is because the ladder was faulty, the driver had fallen asleep, and so forth. But why did this accident happen to me, now? To give an answer to that question is far more difficult and complex. Indeed, the question 'why?' may not be the appropriate question at all.

What is looked for here is a way of understanding what a

certain event – a loss or bereavement – means to our life. A loss has caused a wound. It has taken away part of our life, and we need to adjust to life without this part. A re-alignment has to take place. This means questioning the values which had held true until now, and considering the values which may need to figure more strongly from now on. This is not the same process as finding the practical answer to a question. When people do think it is, then they are into retribution: finding blame and making the guilty party pay. This is often a necessary step in the process of adjustment, but it is not usually the most important step.

The question 'what is the meaning of it?' addresses the person, not just the event. It addresses the life of that person, not just a particular part of it.

There would be little point in asking someone for the story of what happened if there were not the hope or prospect of gaining some insight, and being helped by the telling of the story. Helping a person emotionally does not simply mean hearing a story, but it means helping the person to relate the story – the experience – to the rest of life. Therefore the question 'what is happening?' has to be followed with a question about the meaning of the story.

When we hear someone's story of a bereavement we will undoubtedly be hearing much detail of suffering, caring, pain and love. Some of this may be said to give the story a frame and a place in history. But some of the detail may point to the more intangible, the relationship, to hopes shared and shattered, and to anguish lived through together, and now having to be lived alone. The relationship between parents and children is perhaps the most difficult of all relationships to understand. Children and parents cannot choose each other. Children are a part of their parents, but parents have to bring up children in such a way that they will eventually be independent of them and even to a degree reject the parents and their ways. Parents have to care for their children for about 20 years of their lives, and very likely children have to care for their parents for about 20 years, too. The reversal of the parenting role is often fraught with problems.

What, then, does it mean to lose a parent? This question is not specific to this situation, and should be considered in all helping relationships; it is used specifically here to consider this aspect of loss and grief.

For Audrey, in the scenario at the beginning of the chapter, losing her mother began with a jolt with the positive ultrasound result. Faced with the prospect that the mother would not have much longer to live, Audrey and she set about putting their relationship right. The priority at that stage was not 'getting better', but 'getting it right'.

Audrey had many difficulties in her earlier life, and had also had much help from various types of therapists. But at this stage there was no need of any therapist. Perhaps with all that she had learned earlier but had not been able to apply well then, she had still learned enough to be her own therapist now. This is what helping and counselling is ideally aiming for. Sometimes it takes rather a long time to become evident.

As Audrey had trained as a physiotherapist in the past, she was able to find employment as an assistant in her field after the death of her mother. Her employment record for the few years before then was not good, and so her colleagues may have wondered how it would work out this time. And one can imagine that Audrey bent the ears of her colleagues on many occasions. She was herself in a 'good place' as she called it, but she will still have had to make many connections with her life before and after her mother's death.

Audrey's father had died many years ago and he seemed to have slipped into the background of her memories to such an extent that she remembered little about him. The death of her mother was therefore *the* important death of a parent. This is perhaps unusual. The first parent to die will normally evoke sentiments of primordial attachment and detachment. Love and hate may mingle very strongly in a son or daughter after the death of a parent. Parents who have created a child now make that child wonder, 'what for?' What is the purpose of life? Have the parents given the child a purpose? And if so, is the child fulfilling it? If not, what is either preventing the purpose from being fulfilled, or what is the reason that it is not possible or feasible to fulfil it?

These very basic questions concerning our existence cannot and may not need to be addressed often. They usually only become evident with a major and unexpected event. Had Audrey's mother been ill for a long time and had the two women had time to talk with each other slowly and gently, a process of adaptation would probably have taken place. When this is not possible and one is provoked by unforeseen circumstances, then the physical shock may also call forth the other aspects of the person: the psychological, emotional and spiritual. All aspects of the person are affected by a loss, and all need to adjust to the new circumstances. We can adapt physically much more readily than emotionally; hence the question for the meaning of an event is so vital.

The question does not have to be asked in these particular words; indeed, it may not have to be asked at all. With experience we all recognize when someone is talking about meaningful aspects, or is making allusions to deeper and inner parts of living. If so, this needs to be fostered by being acknowledged and responded to.

Just as the question 'what is happening?' is so fundamental to helping that it is often overlooked, so the question 'what is the meaning of it?' is so fundamental that it is often left out. In my counselling work I have again and again been surprised, when asking this question, that people are astonished – almost always happily so – to be asked this question. It seems often to be the key question, and people are surprised that they had never been asked it before. Such is the make-up of the human being that we often do not tumble to the obvious ourselves, and therefore we may never have asked the question ourselves. But when someone else asks it, it is clear that it is this which will help to unravel the problem.

The question should not be asked too early or too easily in a helping situation. There is a sense in which the moment has to be right for this question to be heard and taken in. But it is also clear that without this question – or some similar way of gaining access to insights – the person cannot move forward. Loss and bereavement are situations where it is easy to become stuck and be dominated by guilt, fear and anger, and the necessary adjustment is not made. This can then lead to physical and emotional pathology. As helpers we do have a responsibility to do what we can to help effectively, and this may be one such way of helping.

But as with this model generally, and with all helping models, the process is not always simple and straightforward. 'What is the meaning of it?' may have to be asked many times, just as the other questions may need repetition. A person may not hear the question, even though it may have been asked several times already. What matters is that we respond to the *person* each time, not to the problem.

The meaning of it

The meaning of a loss, especially of a person, is intensely individual. No two relationships are the same, therefore no two losses are the same. If they were, grieving would not be so difficult. It has also been my experience that if ever I thought I had guessed what the meaning of something would be for a person, I have almost always been wrong. This may not simply mean that I am a bad judge of people, but may also point to the fact that in the last analysis, we are individual and alone. Even though we are constantly with people, there are certain things which we have to do alone. Perhaps deciding what is the meaning of our life, and death, are those two things. Even though we are born in and into at least one relationship, sooner or later that bond has to be broken. Just as the physical umbilical cord has to be cut, so the emotional cord has to be cut in order to live as a human being. When a parent dies, this is made clear beyond doubt. It is often also the first realization of that fact, and it may be difficult to admit this when one is 50, 60 ... .

It is not feasible to ask young children what the meaning is of the loss of a parent. They have their own interpretation, and that should be acknowledged and worked with, but the question as such is not relevant in the same way. It may however be very pertinent to ask it of adolescents who have lost parents, as adolescence is in itself a time of loss and adjustment. Indeed, adults who mourn the death of a parent may be thrown back in memory to adolescence as the last time in which they had 'lost' something significant.

Every important loss brings to the surface other losses experienced. It may be that such losses have not been worked through sufficiently for various reasons. When searching for the meaning of the present loss, it is therefore possible that the meaning is to uncover the earlier loss and understand it better.

Sometimes it is a quite insignificant present loss which brings to mind an important earlier one; sometimes the opposite is true and a present, seemingly important loss, like the death of a parent, may recall an earlier loss which seems trivial. But it is also that earlier losses are not so much events in history as stages of life.

Children who have not experienced a real childhood may become aware of this only in later life and after the loss of a person. It may be that children may have had to look after a sick parent, thus being 'robbed' of an expectation of childhood. It may be that children of one-parent families feel that they have been deprived of a parent figure and image. This could very easily have been the case with Beth and her siblings. In an effort to compensate for this loss they may have wanted to be with their mother all the more and may therefore have suffered other deprivations, such as adequate help and care. Not only will they have lost their mother as well now, but they will also have lost a certain ideal of life. They are therefore not just bereaved of parents, but also of expectations and rewards.

Any significant loss is experienced as a bereavement. When we therefore ask for the meaning of that loss, we may also find that some people have never considered having a meaning in or of their lives. Some people might therefore experience such a question as shocking and painful. For this reason it is imperative that we listen to the client or patient, and in the most skilled way possible use language which is suitable and understandable. This may mean asking gently and only gradually more directly, perhaps using questions like the following:

Do you see any reason behind this?
What connections do you make with other events in your life?
What do you read into the event?
What is important for you in this?

These and similar questions help not only to focus the person's mind, but also to elicit a story. It is important to *ask* the person for his or her own story, not to assume that we know the story, or even to put words into their mouths. This is why this model is based on questions.

It is also important to be very aware that as helpers we cannot give or offer people any meaning. Indeed, the meaning in life is not something manufactured. We discover meaning when we confront the events which happen in our lives. We can create many situations in life and they make us feel good and powerful. But what really shapes our character is what we make of the events which are given to us unbidden. Life is full of these events. How we respond to them shows up our character.

One of the difficulties for many people is the way in which we fight such unbidden events and situations. We resist intrusions into our lives which would disrupt life. We fight illness and old age, and to some extent this is very legitimate. But the balance between resistance and acceptance has constantly to be found again. The meaning of it is expressed in the balance which we create.

Many people express the meaning of death in religious or spiritual terms. Does death have any meaning at all? History shows clearly enough that people have always wrestled with the problem of death. Some of the world's greatest monuments were built in honour of the dead, often implying a hope or belief in an afterlife. It is particularly around the issue of death that religion has always been very influential. Most religions teach that life is not the end, and when life has been taken away, then a belief in a continuing life is important. But as this life has become ever better, so the claims of many religions that the afterlife is worth striving for becomes less credible. It is perhaps only when people have experienced the death of a close person, or have been close to death themselves, that thoughts and assertions about afterlife become meaningful. When we therefore ask the bereaved for the meaning of their lives, it is quite possible that they may now consider the meaning of their lives to be in relation to something beyond rational understanding. As helpers we need to be comfortable with expressions of religious language and practice.

Death – and any important loss – brings us to the realization that our life is finite and that we have to live within the boundaries of finiteness. We cannot recall a dead person to life; we cannot halt the ageing process completely; we cannot stop the clock; we cannot bring back a time of innocence. It tends to be in this crucible of wants and needs and inabilities that we are formed as persons. Perhaps helping someone to find a meaning in doubt, chaos and loss is one of the most significant ways of helping.

Further reading   Ainley, R. (ed.) (1994) *Death of a Mother; Daughters' Stories.* London: Pandora.

Chick, S. (1989) *I Never Told Her I Loved Her.* London: The Women's Press Ltd.

Lindsay, B. and Elsegood, J. (1996) *Working with Children in Grief and Loss.* London: Baillière Tindall.

Oswin, M. (1991) *Am I Allowed to Cry?; A Study of Bereavement Amongst People Who Have Learning Difficulties.* London: Souvenir Press.

Wilson, J. (1989) *Falling Apart.* London: Lions Tracks (Harper Collins).

CHAPTER FOUR

Loss of a child
What is your goal?

Pat and Robin had already three children when Pat found that she was pregnant again. Although it was not a planned pregnancy, she was delighted to have another child, and her family were pleased with her. There was Edward, aged nine, Lucy, aged seven, and five-year-old Alex: old enough to understand but young enough to still form one group.

They were a happy family, all said and done, and Anna, the youngest, was particularly lively. Needless to say she got spoiled by her brothers and sister, but it was all taken in good faith. They all did well at school and all the older ones had gone to university.

Before Anna started at university herself she wanted to have a party to celebrate with friends and acquaintances. Pat and Robin had arranged leaving parties for the other children too, so they joked now that this would be the last one. They hired a hall and prepared everything themselves. They knew the names of all the people who had been invited and had ensured that only limited amounts of alcohol were available.

At some stage Anna said to one of her friends that she was feeling somewhat odd and went to the toilet, presumably to be sick. When she came back she had just time to tell her friend that she had taken an Ecstasy tablet before she collapsed. She was rushed to hospital where she died three days later.

That night Alex disappeared and was found drowned in a canal not very far away. A note on his body simply said that he had given Anna the tablet. At post-mortem it was found that he had also taken some himself.

Christmas Puddings

This year, on the sixteenth anniversary of my first daughter's birth and her brief, three-day life, I felt peaceful and somewhat sad – an *appropriate emotion. Previously I'd busied myself making wonderful Christmas puddings, steaming the house from top to bottom and generally over-occupying my hands so that my mind would not become too grief stricken. I had always dealt with all the aspects of my grief as best I could but always, each year at some point, quite unpredictably around the pertinent dates, I would become overwhelmed with sadness, becoming depressed, and I would relive the trauma of all those events. I'd come to believe that I was to carry around with me a permanent hatred of the autumn, dreading November in particular, when my emotions became numb. I had sudden outbursts of tears and I went around looking grey and drawn for days on end.*

Last year, purely by chance, on Sarah's birthday I was able to use a 'therapeutic technique' as a means of exploring my emotions in a fresh way. It hadn't occurred to me that I still had work to do in this area; I simply felt that I'd already done all that I could. I only mentioned the coincidence in passing and was unsure there might be any value in pursuing it any further. I found myself transported back fifteen years in a very safe, supportive way. I felt able to hold my baby for the first time. I was enabled to talk to her about the confused feelings that I had experienced, and the fact that we were removed from the high-tech neo-natal unit eventually led to that peace.

The whole event was incredibly traumatic and yet at some levels I was stunned by the simplicity of what I was doing and yet knew that it would have a profound effect on me. Hardly daring to believe that there could be any long-term effect, I waited for her birthday to come around. November started and my life carried on peacefully. The anxiety did not increase, I felt more relaxed and had colour in my cheeks. Her birthday itself came and I plodded around in my head. I didn't find any experiences were too much for me to handle – sure I was sad, but not disproportionately so. On the day that she died, I treated myself to a very expensive bouquet of flowers, wept, felt somewhat alone and rather subdued, but incredibly peaceful and I grieved for her appropriately on her anniversary, and I was with that peace. I think this year we may have to buy Christmas puddings from the shop. (G.M.)

'What a waste of a life' is a common expression on hearing of the death of a child. We are confronted with ourselves to a greater extent when we hear of the death of child than of an old person. To the families concerned there is clearly no comparison. Leavitt (1996) makes an interesting observation:

Nurses ... who have had years of experience with dying patients, or with deformed neonates who are on this earth for just a few hours, often wonder whether life has a deeper meaning than what appears to the eye. Particularly interesting is the idea, found in sources as far apart as Jewish Kabbalah and East Asian mysticism, that a soul is sent to this world to undergo a certain 'correction', an experience necessary to its path to perfection. Once this 'correction' has taken place, sometimes after a brief life and sometimes after a long one, the soul returns to the upper worlds. This might give meaning to medical treatment that many would call 'futile'. This philosophy must not be either accepted or rejected dogmatically. Bioethics must investigate it open-mindedly and seriously. Nurses, with much experience of life and death, may be the appropriate people to investigate it.

Neonatal deaths

There is no bigger anticlimax than the birth of a dead baby (Bryan, 1992). Perhaps this is still an understatement.

Stillbirth

Stillbirths (any baby born after 24 completed weeks gestation who shows no sign of life), perinatal deaths (babies stillborn or who die in the first week of life) and neonatal deaths (babies who have shown any signs of life and who die up to the age of 28 days) (Stewart and Dent, 1994, p. 52) account thankfully for very few deaths in the UK. This is far from universal. Birth is a traumatic experience for a baby and it is not surprising therefore that the first weeks and months of life are the most vulnerable.

Intrauterine death may happen at any stage of pregnancy, but it is more noticeable towards the end of the pregnancy. If fetal death has been confirmed, labour is usually induced quickly. There is a sad irony in having to go through the pain and work of labour to produce a dead body. That that body is also one's baby, one's child who had been alive, is therefore devastating, and may remain a devastating memory.

It has now been generally recognized that parents need to see, feel and handle their stillborn baby. Only in this way can they realize both the birth and the death of their baby. The parents have never known the baby alive, but they have been very much aware of it being alive during the pregnancy. Now they must look at it in order to know it. Despite being given time to hold and handle their baby, this is for a relatively short time compared with other events. It is therefore customary in many neonatal units and hospitals to take photographs of the baby and give these to the parents.

Bryan (1992), writing about the loss of a twin at birth, says that '(i)t has only recently been recognised that twin conceptions are much commoner than once thought, but that a large proportion of twin conceptions results in a singleton birth'. Giving birth to twins, one alive and one dead, is focusing on the duality of birth and death even more strongly. It is not surprising that family, friends and health care staff focus on the live child, but the parents may want to grieve for the dead one. The conflicting needs and emotions may be difficult to reconcile.

Perinatal death

Parents of babies who die at or soon after birth find that one of the most hurtful things which people can say to them is, 'you can have another one'. While this is true, such a remark seems to imply that the baby who has died was perhaps not worth living, did not really have a life, or should be replaced quickly so as not to be remembered. But a mother who has been carrying a child for nine months has for that time been in intimate contact with that child and has given of her own life to sustain the growing life. Such a child may also have personified many hopes and expectations of its parents. A time of grieving is therefore as necessary as for any other bereavement. The story at the beginning of the chapter shows this very clearly.

Sudden infant death syndrome (SIDS; cot deaths) is indeed *Every Mother's Nightmare*, as the title of a television documentary shown on ITV, 31 October 1991, suggested. As more becomes known about the syndrome, more fingers may be pointed at parents whose baby dies of SIDS. Parents may be going through their own painful inquisition and having friends and acquaintances make insensitive suggestions can be hurtful in the extreme. A listening ear may be more appropriate at such a time than giving one's own opinions.

Loss of a small child

The difference between an expected and an unexpected death in a child is very similar to that of an adult. But the impact always seems to be deeper because it does not seem 'right' that a child should die. Parents are also responsible for their children, and particularly when a death is unexpected, there is necessarily a sense of guilt present. There may be nothing unusual in leaving a child unattended, or in the care of siblings, or expect that the child can look after himself or herself, but the one time when something happens it will always be seen as having been wrong (Stewart and Dent, 1994, p. 78).

In the UK there have been some tragic events in which children have been killed in recent years. In 1993 Jamie Bulger, a toddler, was killed by two ten-year-old boys. And in 1996, in Dunblane, Scotland, sixteen five- and six-year-old children – half the class – were killed at their school by a gunman. These deaths have affected the whole nation, and have been news the world over. The circumstances of their deaths have not only been cruel and shocking, but senseless. The parents and acquaintances have their own grieving to do, but all of us are addressed by such events. We recognize the killer in us, the person who is capable of revenge, who is mad, cannot stop, or is afraid to stop. It is this which makes such events so poignant. In such circumstances we understand clearly the well-known quote: 'never send to know for whom the bell toll; it tolls for thee' (John Donne, 1624).

We cannot make sense of such events for the people affected directly, but our own contribution to the deaths will make a difference to the whole understanding of grief, living and dying. We may be more empathic when helping people with their losses and griefs because we have faced ourselves in such circumstances.

Adoption

With the availability of birth control and the more ready acceptance of one-parent families, adoption is not very common. Adoption now happens more with older children, those who are handicapped, and children from overseas (Stewart and Dent, 1994, p. 118). Raphael (1984, p. 254) makes the point that the real baby may be very different from the fantasy baby. Despite scans and good antenatal care, some babies are born handicapped, and a mother may reject such a baby. Other mothers decide from early in the pregnancy that the child should be placed for adoption. When that time comes, it may however be very difficult for the mother to give up the child *and* the feelings which went with it. This is almost impossible, as testimonials in fiction and non-fiction have only too clearly pointed out. Indeed, Stewart and Dent (1994, p. 119) give an account of a mother who gave her baby up for adoption. Nobody talked with her about it; she started taking drugs within weeks and continued to do so for years.

It is perhaps even more to difficult to grieve for someone

one knows to be alive still than for someone who has died. Fantasies of meeting the child, of wondering what the child looks like, where he or she is and what they do can be very strong. The child has the possibility to contact the birth mother, but the mother does not have this possibility, so a mother may literally wait for a call which may just as surely never come. Because feelings of loss and grief are not talked about, it does not mean that they do not exist.

When an adopted child does trace the birth mother, the adoptive mother may go through a new and perhaps different kind of grieving. The old wound about possibly not being able to have a child may be opened, but now there may be a sense of being rejected by the adopted child. The 'fantasy' child did not turn out to be what was hoped for, and the child which she had now turns against her.

When health care professionals meet patients and clients, they may come across someone who might be particularly distressed, and on probing just a little further, may discover that this person may be grieving not for the present loss, but for something or someone in the past. The story of the 'Christmas puddings' (p. 36) shows that some unresolved grief may last a very long time (16 years in this case), and had there not been the opportunity to resolve it, it might have gone on for longer still. Time alone will not take the hurt away; talking and sharing may. Being aware of the impact and reality of such losses will certainly help us as helpers to be more effective and humane.

Loss of a sibling

Siblings tend to come off worst in a situation where a child dies. When a child has been ill there will also have been the times of caring, worrying and explaining to siblings. They will be particularly affected when all the attention is suddenly given elsewhere and they may consequently be neglected. Parents may have so much worry and anxiety with the sick child that they simply do not have any more time or emotional energy to cope with the other children. They in turn may worry about 'whether their sister or brother will get better, whether the illness is contagious, whether their own needs will still be met in the family' (Rosen, 1986, p. 60). Rosen also found that siblings 'revealed fear of and preoccupation with needles and other related medical procedures and the physical changes observed in their siblings as a result of treatment. They also ... felt lonely and isolated' (p. 60). If the sibling dies, the parents may then feel that, having neglected their other children, those children may have turned away from them to seek support and comfort elsewhere, and they may in a sense have 'lost' those children too. It is almost as if in such a situation it is impossible to get it right, and this may be a heavy weight on such a family for a long time.

When families split up and re-form, there is also the grief of known patterns and friends. A new family may take on children from an earlier family, and if a child from the other half becomes ill or dies, rivalries and jealousies may arise which may leave children damaged and hurt.

Loss of an adult child

With longer life expectancies it will be increasingly common that older parents may see their adult children die. With smaller families this may be an even harder prospect. Accidents cannot be prevented completely, and AIDS has recently caused many deaths among young adults. While large-scale wars have taken away many sons in the past, this is less common now, but memories of such events are still alive, and the troubles in Northern Ireland have until recently cost many lives on both sides.

Elderly parents whose adult sons or daughters die may feel that they should have died instead. The parents may now have to take over the care of young children and be thrown into a much more active life than they had envisaged. They may feel resentment at this and not have enough energy or resources for this task. Thus they may not have time and space to grieve adequately and grief may therefore be prolonged. On the other hand they may also find a new role in life and put all their energy into caring for the young children, drowning their grief in the care.

Losing an adult child may also happen through other circumstances: children getting married, moving to distant parts of the world, joining strict and exclusive religious groups, or being imprisoned.

Parents may also have excluded their own children themselves, often for ideological or moral reasons. This may be very hard later on for parents who may then not know how to get in touch again with their children if they have changed their minds. This may also be hard for the children concerned and may be a source of constant sorrow.

What is your goal?

The questions 'what is happening?' and 'what is the meaning of it?' equally apply in the situations discussed in this chapter, but the emphasis here will be on the further question 'what is your goal?'.

Helping someone is always done with the aim of leaving the person in a better space than the present. A problem only exists because the person cannot – for whatever reason – make some change or move forward or outward from some morass. As helpers – in whatever capacity – we cannot drag people away or out of some emotional ditch, but by being with them, listening to them and hearing the story, we can perhaps enable them to get to this point themselves.

Being stuck in some emotion or memory is a very human predicament. There is nothing intrinsically 'wrong' or 'bad' about it; very likely it is a defence mechanism for someone in order to cope with a hostile world. The world of the present may not be particularly hostile at all, but earlier events have left marks on the person's psyche which even now react to similar events in ways which were adequate then, but are no longer so. Grieving is one such way of behaving. The mother in the 'Christmas puddings' story demonstrated this well.

Asked if they may want to change, many bereaved people would probably answer yes. They realize that constant grieving is sapping their energy and depriving them of joy. But they would not know how to change. Even if asked the question, 'what is your goal?' they may not know how to answer. The question can really only be asked *after* the question for the meaning has been asked and answered. When the meaning of something becomes evident, then a goal will often present itself quite naturally.

The following quote is not directly related to bereavement, but shows the aspects of meaning and goal well:

An eighty-five-year-old woman from the hillcountry of Kentucky ... was asked to look back over her life and reflect on what she had learned. With that touch of wistfulness that inevitably accompanies any statement beginning 'If I had to do it over...' she said 'If I had my life to live over, I would dare to make more mistakes next time. I would relax. I would be sillier, I would take fewer things seriously ... I would eat more ice cream and less beans. I would perhaps have more actual troubles but fewer imaginary ones. You see, I'm one of those people who lived seriously and sanely hour after hour, day after day. I've been one of those persons who never went anyplace without a thermometer, a hot water bottle, a raincoat, and a parachute. If I had it to do again, I'd travel lighter' (Kushner, 1986, pp. 144–5).

Presumably for this woman the meaning which had emerged was that life was to be enjoyed, not just endured. Therefore her goal is to 'travel lighter'.

This is not meant to imply that grief should not be taken seriously; on the contrary, grief *is* serious, *but it is not all there is to life*.

Any bereaved person is shocked, however little. In physical shock there is a shut-down of non-essential functioning in order to preserve life, and a similar process takes place in emotional shock: everything except the necessary is shut down. But unlike physical shock, the emotional shock is not predictable and people may 'shut down' different functions. When the period of shock wears off, however, they may not be in touch with emotions which are helpful and which are not. Better therefore to stay where they are, emotionally, and not face any of them. This can then easily become a pattern and a pathology results which is subtle but crippling.

For other people, emerging from the shock means going through a time of turbulence, moving in and out of emotional stability. They find themselves in the stage of ambivalence (Kübler-Ross, 1969) or developing awareness (Speck, 1978) or are, according to Worden (1991), working through the task of adjusting to an environment in which the deceased is missing. If the question 'what is your goal?' is asked at such a time, there may be no one clear answer. It may be that one day the goal for a person is to find a new life, and another day the goal might be to be as close as possible to the deceased so as to treasure the memory. This should certainly be respected as a vital part of the adjustment to be made in the initial stages.

Sometimes helpers have a tendency to assume that a person wants to change. After all, helping exists to make the other person feel better. But with assumptions we do not get very far. Indeed, the idea of having a model for helping consisting of questions is precisely in order to hear what the other has to say. The question, 'what is your goal?' is indeed a very clear question looking for a clear answer, but the answer may be 'not to have a goal', or 'staying where I am'. The question 'what is your goal?' is only valid when the other two questions have been asked and answered. If we jump in too quickly with ideas of goals, we may be rebuffed and may have done harm rather than good.

Nurses in particular, but helpers generally, like to see results and have an answer to any difficulty. It may therefore be going against the grain to sit and wait, stand by almost helpless while a person struggles, and perhaps watch someone make a mistake. Helping, however, is not 'taking over', but *helping* the other person to find her or his own way, work through problems, and come out stronger.

As with the question 'what is the meaning of it?' the question 'what is your goal?' is a very individual thing. As helpers we may have our own ideas of what someone's goal might be, but we cannot impose it. We may be able to make suggestions in order to help the person to focus, but these are and must be suggestions and pointers. Sometimes such suggestions will help the person to see a way forward.

Very often when I use this question people are not at all sure what they might answer. If I then say, for instance

You may want to invite friends more? or
Could you now go on that holiday?

the answer comes back, 'No, I will start with the driving lessons'. Having proposed some possibilities, the person is helped to focus on her or his own needs.

In the course of a conversation we often hear important words or phrases which can be captured and perhaps reflected back to the person. When we allow a person to express herself or himself openly, then that person will probably – even without any particular help – talk about meanings and significance and goals and aims, hopes and desires. This may be done without the person being aware of it. But if our quality of listening is good, then we will hear such words and expressions and present them back to the person as their own 'work'. They may be surprised that what they have actually said is the right thing. It is only 'right' because it is suited to that person.

'What is your goal?' need not be asked in this particular way; indeed, it may not have to asked at all. But the direction of a conversation should be that at the end the person is in a better space than at the beginning. If not, we have not been helpful. Even having a good moan, when no particular outcome is sought, can be good, if a goal is to let off steam, let go of unnecessary feelings and pent-up emotions, and if this frees a person to go on.

The goals of helping

When considering helping a bereaved person, it may be tempting to have a checklist and imagine that the person needs to achieve this or that. Or, like the nurse who wrote that she and all her 'set' were taught about the grieving process, and would probably 'still, more than a decade later, reel off Kübler-Ross's stages without having to think about it and ... what to say and what not to say to the person who had just lost a loved one' (Anonymous, 1993). It is not *what* we say or do which counts so much as *how* we say and do something. We can say all the right things, but if they are not said with actual conviction and integrity, then they are not only not worth anything, but are hurtful. And at crucial moments we hear selectively: we hear what we want to hear, good or bad.

Worden (1991, p. 80) says that '(t)he goal of grief therapy is to resolve the conflicts of separation and to facilitate the completion of the grief tasks'. When thinking of goals it may be useful to think of different types of goals: short-, medium- and long-term goals. They may be different and emerge one after the other, or there may be one or two clear long-term goals, and a few short-term goals to achieve quickly.

Many people feel that in the first weeks after a bereavement they are happier with very clear and specific tasks to do and achieve. The various arrangements which have to be made after a death focus a person often in very helpful ways. But after that there have to be other tasks, too. Having to see to financial affairs, rearranging rooms and cupboards are also important. In doing such tasks the bereaved is in a way separating herself or himself from the dead person in a very practical way. By changing the surroundings we acknowledge that life continues. Some people who find it difficult to make decisions find that mentally asking the dead person for help can focus their thoughts and actions. Most likely the dead person would not want their loved ones to become immobile, but move on as necessary.

What is right for one person may not be right for another. Some people find that they have to clear wardrobes of clothing quickly and others feel that they need to do it gradually; some people feel the need to socialize and be 'merry widows' and other feel that they want to wait.

The people in the stories at the beginning of the chapter have had to think in terms of goals, too, but very differently.

The mother of the baby who died shows a typical reaction of many people: for years the anniversary is a difficult time. Asked what she might see as a goal, she might perhaps have said, 'getting through November every year'. She did not seem aware of the possibility that this might change. But someone or something helped her to change, and she describes this movingly. Her goal on that particular day was to feel good about the day, the memories, and about herself too. And it worked. This is the astonishing thing. It is not astonishing for helpers, because they will have witnessed such changes before; but for the bereaved themselves, it may appear like a miracle – and that is OK.

The parents of the two children who died will have had a very different story to tell. One child, Anna, died because of the thoughtless action of another, Alex, and then he died at his own hands, not able to cope with the consequences of his actions. This is a double tragedy. The parents will have had to work through a great deal of anger: at hearing that their son took and supplied drugs; sorrow: at losing two children at once; guilt: at perhaps not having talked enough with their children about the dangers of drugs, or letting them be too free. Their goals – when they were ready to think in terms of goals – might be to function as a 'new' family unit; come to terms with the fact that they could not have supervised their children constantly, and that their children will have to learn to take responsibility for their own lives.

The grief experienced at the loss of a person from illness or accident is different from that experienced after a suicide. The feelings of guilt in the case of suicide will always be much stronger. For these parents, who are experiencing both types of loss at once, this is a crucial time in their lives and they may need a great deal of help. The siblings, Edward and Lucy, will also have had to work through their grief. They too may feel anger: at being left behind by their brother and sister; sorrow: at losing part of their own lives; and perhaps guilt: at maybe having taken each other too much for granted, showing off their prowess in front of the younger ones and perhaps goading them on to dare trying drugs. But their feelings of guilt may be less obvious and perhaps less strong, though that may be conjecture. They too may need much help and sensitive listening.

It may be that nurses and other health care workers come in touch with one or other of the persons described in these stories much later in life, when they are ill or perhaps in hospital. At that time they may not be actively grieving for the people described, but they may be having a difficult time coming to terms with a present illness. It may then be that asking 'what is happening?' may bring to light old wounds, unhealed or newly opened. When then further asking 'what is your goal?' the answer may be, 'getting through the present difficulties'. This may seem strange, when really the old wounds may seem a great deal more raw and painful than the present ones. It is not easy to go into detail over something which may have happened a long time ago. On the other hand, dealing effectively with the present may also help to clear up the past.

But the converse may also be the case: dealing with the old wounds may also deal with the present ones. This may be just the reverse of the earlier scenario, and may sound contradictory. But in helping we have to live with contradictions. They are only contradictions if we label them as such. In real life it simply means that every person is different. Listening to the person we hear his or her story – not ours – and that is the story which counts.

Further reading

Allende, I. (1995) *Paula*. London: Flamingo.

Fraser, M. (1984) *Beyond the Rainbow*. London: Lions.

Hill, S. (1986) *In the Springtime of the Year*. Harmondsworth: Penguin.

McEwen, I. (1987) *The Child in Time*. London: Picador.

Sourkes, B.M. (1996) *Armfuls of Time; The Psychological Experience of the Child with a Life-Threatening Illness*. London: Routledge.

Walterstorff, N. (1987) *Lament for a Son*. Sevenoaks: Hodder and Stoughton.

Videos

When Our Baby Died (a video about grief for parents and families).

Grieving After the Death of Your Baby (book accompanying the above video).

Death at Birth (training video for health care professionals).

All available from: Professional Care Productions Ltd, 1 Millside, Riversdale, Bourne End, Bucks SL8 5EB, UK.

CHAPTER FIVE

Abortion and miscarriage
How are you going to do it?

....

Carlie was 16 when she found that she was pregnant. She and Mark had been going steady for a good few months when he began to pressure her to have sex. Although reluctant at first, Carlie was nevertheless excited as she and her friends had discussed having sex often; now she would be joining the 'other' group: those who could talk from experience. Carlie had bought a packet of condoms, but on the night Mark was adamant that he would not use one. Sex was not sex with a condom. Carlie was concerned not to lose Mark and so she gave in. She was horrified to find that she was pregnant.

She knew that she could not tell her mother of the pregnancy, so she talked to an unmarried aunt of whom she was quite fond. Although the aunt was kind, she did not give Carlie any option, but phoned up a clinic there and then and made an appointment. Carlie knew that an abortion was the only rational way, but she also felt hesitant. She knew that she was able to give consent for the abortion on her own and that her mother would never need to know, but when the day came, she was not happy. It was all over easily and quickly and she had managed to hide it successfully from her mother.

The next hurdle was if to tell Mark or not. Carlie felt strongly that it was his baby, too. But she could not bring herself to tell him. Instead, she got pregnant again by him just a few weeks later. This time she told her mother, also telling her that she had already made enquiries and knew of a clinic. She had another abortion, this time it fell in school holidays. Again, she could not bring herself to tell Mark, but now she felt so bad about it, she broke off with him. He called her a few names and then just went his way.

Three years later she got married and was convinced that everything was going to work well: Barry and she were very much in love and wanting a family. But Carlie found that she could not get pregnant. When some investigations were carried out it soon became clear why. When she told Barry of the reason, he could not take it and left her there and then. Her life seemed ruined and shattered.

Daniel and Terry had two girls aged six and four and secretly they longed to have a boy. They had tried for a long time when Terry found that she was pregnant again. The evening when she told Daniel she had arranged a special dinner for themselves and had bought a rather expensive bottle of wine. They were very excited. What was more, the expected date was actually her own birthday!

But then it happened: Terry had a miscarriage when she was 14 weeks pregnant. She was devastated; her birthday would be tinged with sadness. She really grieved, and although only a few people knew that she had a miscarriage, she could not tell even those people what were the reasons for her depressions. Another miscarriage some time later made her realize that her dream of a third child might not come true, but it did – 10 years later and very unexpectedly. And it was a boy.

Abortion and miscarriage are opposites in the spectrum of reasons for a pregnancy to be interrupted. But they are put together in this chapter because some of the after-effects of both abortion and miscarriage can be quite similar.

It is now clear that up to 80% of pregnancies actually end in miscarriage (Oakley *et al.*, 1984, p. 115), but that women are often not aware of this. But abortion is a self-chosen ending of pregnancy which is surrounded with much emotive language which does not apply to miscarriage, nor to any of the other aspects of loss and death considered in this book.

Abortion

In her ground-breaking work on women's moral development *In a Different Voice*, Gilligan (1982) describes her work with women who had abortions. This led her to put forward the theory that women are more concerned with relationships and with care than with justice. Being concerned about relationships then also led women to consider their responsibilities. She uses the example of Jake and Amy, two 11-year old children, to measure their moral development. Thus,

(t)o Jake, responsibility means not doing *what he wants because he is thinking of others; to Amy, it means* doing *what others are counting on her to do regardless of what she herself wants. Both children are concerned with avoiding hurt but construe the problem in different ways – he seeing hurt to arise from the expression of aggression, she from a failure of response* (p. 38).

This extract mirrors closely the story of Carlie, her boyfriend and also her husband Barry, and of countless other similar stories. Carlie was concerned not to cause harm: to her boyfriend, her mother and her aunt, and in the process she is *doing* what in fact harms her.

Carlie told her story to a student nurse at the admission interview. The student recognized Carlie's feelings and asked her if she would consider counselling to help her with her feelings of ruin and guilt. Carlie was hesitant because she felt that she could not trust anyone to take her seriously. Her mother, aunt, boyfriend and clinic staff had all made her do things which she had not wanted to do, but nobody had heard her silent cries. The student nurse said that she was not a counsellor, but might have some experience which might be of help. When the two were alone together, the student admitted that she also had an abortion some years ago, and together they explored their feelings and so helped each other.

Laurent (1991) says that

women seeking advice about an unwanted pregnancy are at the mercy of the moral judgements of whichever professional they turn to. Abortion is such an emotive issue that it seems many health professionals direct women, however unconsciously, along the lines they consider right, rather than letting the woman herself decide. Who a woman turns to depends on what is available in her area. Whether she receives counselling depends on the qualifications of the person she sees.

Blain (1993) too, reports that some hospital nurses hold unkind and punitive attitudes towards women who chose to have abortions. In her study, nurses were particularly low on empathy, and for this she adds a note of reflection: 'It is perhaps true to say that without the caring aspect of the role, a nurse becomes nothing more than a skilled technician or even a general "dogsbody".'

The reasons for the termination of pregnancy are many and varied, but whatever the reasons, there tends to be at least some grieving which may not be entirely resolved. Raphael (1984, p. 239) suggests that women in the 'younger age group (especially first pregnancies), those persuaded to termination by others, those lacking social support, those having it under socially negative or illegal circumstances, are most likely to be at risk' of grieving and mourning. When the termination has also been an attempt to solve a conflict, but which failed to be the solution, then there may be even more risk of long-term grieving.

Abortion is surrounded by emotive language. 'Murder' is often applied to termination of pregnancy, and when a fetus of a few weeks' gestation is referred to as a 'baby' as a matter of course, feelings are inevitably aroused, whatever the argument involved.

Narratives tell of women feeling 'unclean', guilty, 'black and dirty inside' (Raphael, 1984, p. 241), experiencing low self-esteem (Penson, 1990, p. 74) and being protective of their bodies (Speck, 1978, p. 36) and Gilchrist *et al.* (1995) report that '(i)n women with no previous psychiatric history, acts of self-harm were found to be more common in those who either had a termination or who were refused one'.

The fact that an abortion often happens very quickly, and to deal with a present crisis rather than a long-term change, means that there is generally little time beforehand for counselling. Although most pregnancy advice services offer counselling, it may be that at such a time this is not actually easy for the person concerned. Post-abortion counselling may be helpful, but 'women do not tend to seek it' (Worden, 1991, p. 107). Thus they are left with their feelings which then, like all unresolved grief, may become a great burden.

The conflicting feelings around abortion: being glad that a huge problem can be solved easily, and yet feeling guilty about it, may make it difficult to see such feelings in terms of grieving and bereavement. And when using such words, the connection with death may bring up other emotions which may be buried deep in the psyche.

Most family planning and abortion clinics offer post-abortion counselling, but women are very reluctant to seek it (Worden, 1991, p. 107). Because of this, there may be significant grief and anger later on in life, perhaps at the menopause, and this may lead to severe problems. When this may become evident, the person may be greatly helped to work through the grief left over from an abortion.

The role of the father is often disregarded. Men may feel that they have to cheer up their wives or partners, or that they should do this. But they may also feel let down, betrayed and pushed aside. Being perhaps even less able to deal with their feelings, men may lose out greatly in this aspect, and there is therefore an even greater need to listen sensitively and with a non-judgemental ear.

Abortion after diagnosis of a handicapped or unviable fetus is a difficult decision to make for all affected. Counselling will always be offered in these cases and should be done by experienced staff. There may be pressure on the couple to have a termination in order not to bring a handicapped or sick child into the world. But the decision must be the parents' own, and they should be supported in whatever decision they take.

Miscarriage

There is no stigma attached to miscarriage as there is to abortion. Indeed, 'miscarriage', or *spontaneous abortion*, is accepted as a regrettable form of loss of pregnancy which was generally wanted.

Perhaps one of the most widely recognized feelings after miscarriage is the sense of failure as a woman. The idea that a woman is not good enough demonstrates 'the common feeling that the miscarriage is a kind of punishment and is the individual's fault. A series of miscarriages can leave a woman obsessed with the need to have a child' (Penson, 1990, p. 74).

A personal process of enquiry may lead many women and couples to find reasons for a miscarriage, blaming themselves and perhaps each other. Women may blame men for pushing them too hard for sexual relations, and men blaming women for not telling them the truth about past sexual activity. All this may be in an effort to deal with the resultant grief. But this may in fact be due to a sense of helplessness in the face of the grief. Displaced emotions can be a way of seemingly dealing with painful memories.

Dealing with the pain of a miscarriage by trying to replace the lost child with another one may only add to the sense of loss. When the earlier loss has not been acknowledged, then a 'replacement' may only ever be a replacement and not the 'real thing', leaving the grief still unsolved.

Like an abortion, a miscarriage can be hidden, and not many people may know about it. For fear of exposing themselves, women may want to hide their miscarriage and so, sadly, cut themselves off from effective help and support. Women who have had a miscarriage may live through the various stages of the pregnancy, imagining what might have happened at each stage. When they get to the time when the birth should have taken place, they may feel particularly bereft. Again, because the whole event may have been hidden, this may also feel a very lonely time, and acutely painful. Sharing some of the ideas and fantasies may be very helpful.

Raphael (1984, pp. 235–6) mentions fearfulness, sadness, anger, guilt and despair as the main emotions experienced by women who had miscarried. It is not difficult to relate these to the story described above. Terry clearly feared that she might not ever be able to have the boy she wanted. She will have been sad that this should be in her family who had everything to give to a child. She may have been angry that it should have been her, to be in this predicament. And she may very likely have felt guilt at perhaps being 'greedy' in wanting another child, and that not just one, but two miscarriages, were the ways in which she was being punished for her greed and selfishness.

Particularly in the situation of a miscarriage – hidden and lonely as it may be – there may easily be an element of retribution present. We think so often in terms of $1 + 1 = 2$, that is, being selfish or greedy secretly and now being punished for it. This may be one of the reasons why women may behave in ways which please others rather than themselves: not to hurt others. Understanding responsibility may then mean understanding responsibility in terms of self, others and society. This may help to show that in life the events which affect us do not happen in terms of mathematics, but in terms of relationships. This in turn may give a new view of moving forward from ideas and ideals that may be rather stuck.

How are you going to do it?

The earlier questions in this model are the sort of questions which normally elicit a story; this question asks for specific details.

Most of us are aware that knowing that we must do something and actually doing it are two different things. New Year resolutions are notorious for being made but not kept. We know what is good for us, but putting it into practice is not so easy. If it were simply a question of changing a routine it could be done, but here a change of attitude is demanded, and it is this which is difficult.

The three previous questions all help a person to 'find' herself or himself, look at a situation critically, see the wider connections, hear the memories and feelings, and endeavour to make sense of the situation by considering what the meaning or purpose might be of a loss or bereavement (or other event). Each question builds on the other, in order to unravel what might have become a very tight and perhaps painful entity. Asking 'what is the meaning of it?' tries to make sense of the actual circumstances; 'what is your goal?' tries to see the meaning as something which can be transferred into practice;

and 'how are you going to do it?' directs the person into very practical ways of achieving the goals.

Many helpers imagine that when they have helped a person to gain insights they have done their work. Having or gaining insights can be quite disconnected from doing something about it. Many of us know that we must change in many situations, but when the actual situation happens, we don't.

A very common expression is, 'if only ...'. If only she would do it differently, we would all be happy. If only I had enough money. If only he would work with us, all would be well. If only she would stop thinking in this negative way, she would see how good life is. 'If only' is wishful thinking and as such hardly ever comes true. In the very expression 'if only' there is an element of helplessness, which may actually be a defence mechanism for doing something which might be too difficult. Changing an attitude is the ultimate way of being involved with a situation. Changing an attitude affects us personally and directly, and we are often not ready or not willing. We think that others should change, not us.

Another aspect of wishful thinking is that if the other person would change, *our* lives would be better. If we want something to be different or better, *we* have to change; *we* have to make it different. We cannot, as helpers, change a third person. A client who says, 'can you tell my husband to do ...' is deluding herself. A helper who thinks he can counsel a husband via his wife is deluding himself. Hence the question 'how are you going to do it?' is a question directly addressed to the person concerned. It is possible to lay the emphasis on the different words in every question, and here it may therefore often be 'how are *you* going to do it?'

Helping another person means helping that person to take responsibility for her or his thoughts, actions and reactions. It means empowering the other person to take decisions and be responsible for them. To do the work of helping to the end, we have to see the process right through and be assured ourselves that the client or patient has all the means for this empowerment. This includes the last stage of putting insights into action.

These four questions are a model for helping generally. They are not specific to loss and bereavement. But applying the questions to the subject may be best done by applying them to the two stories above. Both stories were related in situations where the main person – Carlie in the story concerning abortions, and Terry in the story concerning miscarriages – met with a nurse some time after the event. It may be that nurses tend to meet such people only some time after the main events occurred. It may only be by listening with empathy to a person that such a story is actually told to a relative stranger.

The question 'how are you going to do it?' needs to address three elements: attention, compassion and forgiveness. These are three words which, like the four questions, I have gleaned from various sources and somehow put together into a model. Like the questions, it may not be the words themselves which are important, but what they convey or signify.

Attention

When the question 'how are you going to do it?' is asked, some people become impatient or dismissive: 'Oh, I know how to do it'. Depending on the context, this may be so. But it can also be a way of saying: don't bother me any more; I cannot cope with more.

When a goal has been reached or elicited, it is very important that it is stated, spelled out and 'captured'. It may not need to be a big goal, but by spelling it out and paying attention to it, it is like a bond between the two people. Saying it to another commits the person to it, and the helper shares by accepting the commitment. If it goes well or badly, the helper has a right to ask how it went. Once spoken, a goal imagined becomes a goal to be achieved.

In the story of Carlie it is possible to imagine many different goals for her. When she told this story to the nurse at the admission interview, the emphasis may have been on the helplessness which Carlie stressed. A goal might therefore be for Carlie to get over the operation for which she was admitted, and then see again what life might hold for her. Or another goal might be to come to terms with the loss of her fertility; or to think what she might need to say early on to a new boyfriend. It is possible to imagine that Carlie might be looking to get away from her sense of rejection. This would be a realistic goal.

How is she going to achieve this goal? The questions asked earlier will have helped her to see many of the issues surrounding her present position. There will have been a lot of attention paid already to various aspects. She should now focus her attention on reaching her goal of not feeling rejected any more. This is clearly a tall order. It may be easier to say 'to feel less rejected' or 'to overcome the sense of rejection'.

This will involve a change of attitude. 'How are you going to do it?' may therefore include some means of overcoming the repeated thoughts or feelings of rejection.

In order to 'anchor' a goal it is useful to think in very practical terms which can be achieved. Overcoming negative thoughts can be helped by consciously acknowledging them each time they occur *without judging them*. This is another form of attention. Negative or painful thoughts are only so because we make them so. Thoughts by themselves are neutral; it is only because we judge and label them that they become 'good' or 'bad'. When they are 'bad' they are so only because we seem to have an inbuilt judge sitting on our shoulders who condemns us constantly. Perhaps this judge has the voice of a parent, or in Carlie's case, her aunt, her boyfriend, or her husband. When the thoughts arise, we need to be aware of the thoughts and the judge, waiting to pounce, but we can stop the judge. This is a change of attitude. We are in control now, not the judge; we allow ourselves to be in control.

This is a very 'conscious' exercise and is quite hard at first. Many people find that they can only do it consciously to some extent. Warning them beforehand may help, and encouraging them during an exercise may be vital. In this example the 'judge' has almost been made into a real person. Sometimes when we can turn a thought into a fact or visualize something in a concrete way, it becomes manageable. This is not possible for everybody, and should not used in an indiscriminate way; it is given as an example here.

The word 'attention' is therefore used with two meanings here: the helper helps the client to focus on the goal by 'concretizing' it; and the client pays attention to the components of the goal, that is, the thoughts which get in the way of living more satisfyingly.

Compassion

Being aware of the thought processes which go on can be very difficult and taxing. It can also be very revealing because this is a new kind of awareness. Some people, imagining the 'judge' as a little person or some goblin or devil or other entity, have found this exercise quite fun. But clearly it is not an end in itself. We help others to be aware of their feelings and thoughts in order that they can move forward. When we have listened enough to our thoughts and are aware of the process by which we allow them, there has to come a time of dealing with them.

Carlie was particularly aware of feelings of rejection. When she has spent some time – perhaps a few days – being aware of herself every time a thought about rejection or feeling of pain of rejection arises, then she needs to consider what to do with the feeling. It is now no longer judged, or at least no longer judged automatically in a bad way. She may begin to see that feeling rejected after her experiences is OK. She has a right to feel like this; maybe she should feel like this; it is not bad to feel like this; this is simply *how* she is feeling. When she can begin to see that her feelings are legitimate, then she begins to see them in a different light. Then she is beginning to treat them with compassion.

Compassion is a word which has been used increasingly frequently. In essence it means 'suffering with', but the way in which the word is used implies more a sense of acceptability, standing by, not rejecting, letting be, respecting. This usually applies to people, but in the example used here it can apply to feelings – or rather to the person who experiences feelings of rejection. When Carlie can be compassionate to herself, she begins to accept herself and then does not need to reject herself any longer. She may then actually see that she only feels rejected because she allowed herself to be rejected. But she does not have to reject herself. If others reject her, that is their problem, and she does not need to take on their problems. She suffers from their inability to handle their own problems, but she does not have to take them on herself. In this way she can learn to accept herself, respect herself and let herself be herself.

Compassion is only one way of describing what is happening. In the language of psychology, words like self-acceptance, being non-judgemental and empathic with oneself would probably come nearest. When using the word compassion I would also include loving oneself as a person, with both one's bright and dark sides. This is a concept which many people have difficulty with. They equate self-love with selfishness. But there is a great difference. Anyone who has been bereaved in whatever way has been wounded and we often have difficulty in accepting ourselves with our wounds. We can do it; we can see both the positive and the negative parts of ourselves and love both parts. Selfishness is exhibiting greed and pride and possessiveness, not seeing the negative aspects of these traits.

When it therefore comes to dealing with the feelings left behind from a loss or bereavement, we have to learn to accept ourselves again, now with the wound. This can be a difficult process. The wound is often so deep that it is feelings like rejection or guilt which are accessible. When dealing with the feelings we may gain access to the wound. It is only when we deal kindly – compassionately – with the feelings that we can get to the wound. This kindness is an expression of self-love, allowing the wound to heal.

Forgiveness

This word, too, can be expressed in different ways. It means a letting-go or giving up.

Carlie, in her quest to feel less rejected, first had to come very close to herself and her feeling, then consider them not as simply 'bad' but as having perhaps protected her at a time of hurt; now she has to let them go. Having recognized the feelings for what they are, that is, like a bandage around the wound, holding it together, she will realize that the wound has now healed and that the bandage is no longer necessary. She will need to let it go.

For some people, such a realization can be a cathartic experience. It may be said here that this is perhaps more what might happen at the time of asking 'what is the meaning of it?', and this is perhaps right. If so, it simply shows that the process of helping and the stages passed through by a client never follow each other so neatly that they do not overlap and interact. Seeing the need to let go of feelings is the last step in this process. But how, practically, is Carlie to do this?

Just as she had been paying attention to her feelings earlier, and then accepting them, so now she has another mental job to do. When the feelings do arise and she recognizes them and does not condemn them, she may now have to use another technique to let them go. She may need to address the feelings in a personal sort of way. She may actually have to say to herself and her feelings, 'Thank you for coming and thank you for being here. You have helped me in the past, but I don't need you any longer. I say good-bye to you'. This is a very graphic way of answering the question 'How are you going to do it?': simply saying 'good-bye', or 'I let you go'. These may not be the right words, but a deliberate and clear way of pushing away and not letting invade again is called for. We all have our own ways of speaking to ourselves. If we have learned anything from compassion, then we can do this letting go in a compassionate way. Some people may be much more forceful and direct and others may be more tentative and polite. As long as the result is a sense of freedom and a new energy, the goal will have been achieved.

This may take quite a long time. Some of our ways of defence against anxiety have been learned and kept over months and years and are therefore ingrained in the psyche. It is not possible to change overnight. If this were to happen we might have caused another wound. But a deliberate working at ourselves and never giving up hope that a change is possible may be the only way forward. This is why it is often so helpful to have someone with whom to discuss these processes and who encourages rather than judges further. The attitude which is needed to want and sustain the change is therefore the operative force. The last effort is always one of letting go in order to be free again for the present.

All the stages of grieving described in Chapter 2 have some form of letting go. Acceptance (Kübler-Ross, 1969), emotionally relocating the deceased and moving on with life (Worden, 1991) and resolution (Speck, 1978) all include or allude to a conscious letting go. I have used the word forgiveness for this because this involves a relationship. We forgive a person. Letting go means letting go of our feelings, guilt or resentments which are normally directed towards the person who died. We need to forgive that person and not hold it against him or her. Most people try to do their best, but they – like us – do not succeed. They did not know how to do better at the time. They have moved on and so have we. It is therefore good to be able to say 'I do not hold it against you'. Forgiveness may not be everybody's favourite word, but most people know what is meant by it. The importance of relationships has been alluded to at the beginning of the chapter, and concluding the process of counselling and helping by mentioning relationships again brings us full circle with the act of forgiveness or letting go.

The example used here has been one of dealing with feelings and emotions left behind as memories. Another form of goal and how to achieve it might have been to consider how Carlie might tell a new boyfriend of her past. This might involve actual scenarios of possibilities. One might have thought of how Daniel could be helped to get in touch with his feelings, needs and desires and thus help Terry to do the same. Equally, all the other stories considered in the other chapters also have to address the question of 'How are you going to do it?' too, sooner or later. Only when this question also has been asked and answered can a helping process really be said to have been successful.

Further reading Andrews, J. (1993) Abortion. In: Tschudin, V. (ed.) *Ethics: Aspects of Nursing Care*. London: Scutari.

Gilligan, C. (1982) *In a Different Voice*. Cambridge, MA: Harvard University Press.

Kohn, I. & Moffitt, P.-L. (1994) *Pregnancy Loss: A Silent Sorrow*. London: Hodder Headline.

Kohner, N. & Henley, A. (1995) *When a Baby Dies: The Experience of Late Miscarriage, Stillbirth and Neonatal Death*. London: Pandora and SANDS (Stillbirth and Neonatal Death Society).

Lachelin, G.C.L. (1996) *Miscarriage; The Facts*. (2nd edn). Oxford: Oxford University Press.

McDonald, M. (1996) *Loss in Pregnancy; Guidelines for Midwives*. London: Baillière Tindall.

Pizer, H. & O'Brien, C. (1980) *Coping with a Miscarriage*. London: Jill Norman.

Rajan, L. & Oakley, A. (1993) No pills for heartache: the importance of social support for women who suffer pregnancy loss. *Journal of Reproductive and Infant Psychology* **11**: 75–87.

CHAPTER SIX

Infertility
Unconditional positive regard

....

James and Heather had now been married for ten years. James had an important job in banking and Heather had a small business as an interior designer. In this capacity she was working at a local GP surgery where she met Denise, the practice nurse.

One day Denise noticed that Heather looked drawn and seemed restless. They got into conversation, and although Heather first denied any problem, she later admitted that she had something which bothered her. Only on the third 'chance' meeting with Heather did Denise hear of the problem of infertility. James had asked Heather not to tell anyone of the 'problem' and not to let anyone know that they were having investigations for infertility. Heather had gone along with this request for years, but now began to find it difficult to hide it even from her mother. She began to feel very alone with her misery. Denise did not want to probe, but Heather seemed to relax when she did talk. In the course of the conversation it emerged that James was also totally against adoption. Heather was very clear that they loved each other deeply and that this was the reason why she had respected James' requests all this time. She admitted to Denise that she would like to talk more, but that she also felt guilty betraying her husband. Denise listened attentively, and Heather even admitted that so far no reason had been found for the infertility. This made the whole situation only worse.

Geraldine and Thomas were both teachers. They had moved to a small village where Thomas had accepted the post of head teacher in the local school. When, after three years of marriage, there was no sign of pregnancy, they both went to have investigations. When this was done, they took several decisions. They decided that they would tell their respective parents and ask them to be open with all their friends and families about their infertility. But they would tell no-

one, not even their parents, which one of them was infertile. This would be their own secret entirely. They had also decided that they would be looking to adopt children from overseas, and finally they had a family of three children, each from a different continent.

Although both Geraldine and Thomas were very happy and contented with their choice, every now and again they found a need to talk with a friend who had become close, and work through different aspects of their 'loss'. The children they had gave them much joy – and plenty of sorrow, too – but the pain of not being quite a 'man' and quite a 'woman' surfaced every now and again, though even the friend never found out which of them was infertile.

Infertility

The problem of infertility is as old as humanity. The Bible recounts several poignant stories of infertility and rites and means for overcoming this. Indeed, the three monotheistic religions, Judaism, Christianity and Islam – often also known as the 'Abrahamic religions' – might not exist in their form today, had Abraham died childless as he thought he would (Genesis 15:2).

Schofield (1995, p. 139) believes that 10 to 15% of all couples are infertile; that 'about half of the couples evaluated and treated in infertility clinics become pregnant'. It is very easy in infertility to concentrate on the problem and the mechanics of infertility and not consider the personal suffering and feelings of the people concerned. Since the investigations in the male partner are relatively easily carried out, it is also possible to overlook a man's emotional needs more easily than a woman's.

With the known declining sperm counts in Western males, this is, however, a problem waiting to become a serious concern for humanity. But no doubt for all concerned it is still a personal tragedy when faced with it. The traditional male roles are changing, and many men now find that when they do show and express feelings they are not as easily and naturally helped as women. Therefore finding themselves infertile can be an enormous challenge to men, physically, emotionally, and in terms of known expectations.

Gould (1993, p. 465) makes the very valid point that 'patients troubled by fertility problems demand considerable sensitivity combined with interpersonal and educative skills'. She goes on to highlight the myths surrounding fertility and its treatments, such as stress causing infertility, or that adopting a child may help a couple to conceive naturally when they are no longer so desperate to have a child.

Harris *et al.* (1991) cite several clients who reported their feelings of loss when they experienced miscarriage after infertility treatment. Because such women will have pregnancy tests rather earlier than usual, they may be aware of a miscarriage, rather than a normal period. Once they knew what they were looking for, they were also literally holding their breath, 'waiting to lose', that is, almost looking out for signs of impending miscarriage. Couples described the 'once-present, but now lost, entity as a baby, an embryo, a pregnancy, a sac, or an egg'. Grieving for such a loss is perhaps difficult, but also necessary. One client remembered that it was a nurse at the clinic who had said to her 'you have miscarried. Let yourself grieve', giving this client an opportunity to see her loss in perspective.

Infertility treatments are often long, intimate, and put strain on a couple by requiring them to monitor details which to other people might seem trivial or private. The possibility that a treatment may not work is always there. And each failed treatment is another disappointment. As well as being uncomfortable, treatments (especially the ovulation stimulating drugs) are never without risk in themselves. If *in vitro* fertilization (IVF) is used, there is a real possibility of multiple births, bringing with it its own problems of possibly having to destroy one or more fetuses, or that the babies born will be premature and therefore more likely to die or be otherwise impaired.

Treatment has come to be seen as the norm when someone is infertile, giving infertility the status of illness. When someone therefore is still unable to maintain a pregnancy even after several treatments, there is always the possible stigma of there being 'something wrong' with the couple. These days it may no longer lead to death, but the reproach may last all the longer.

Adoption is not as easy as it once was, with fewer babies and children abandoned or given away by unmarried mothers. And adoption from other countries or cultures is often frowned upon.

The human race can only be maintained because of procreation, and perhaps a person's deepest longing is to ensure that his or her own creation is continued through children. It is not simply a wish to have a baby because babies are lovely and smell nice; the desire to have a child is the need to maintain life and leave something behind which is distinctly personal.

It is probably true that the more one cannot have something, the more one wants it. Many people regard having children be their 'right'. And this seems to be the implication of being human. But when *claiming* the right to have children, this involves a responsibility by someone else to supply that right. In practice this has often come to mean that solutions to infertility are sought on the basis of demand and supply. Admitting that one cannot have a baby would be admitting failure. Since fertility treatment is less and less often given in NHS-run clinics, clients have to pay, and this can be very costly. It therefore means that only the wealthy can afford it. Those who are not so well off are thus twice stigmatized: being infertile and being poor.

When infertility is established and treatment has not been successful, the time will come for a couple to look the inevitable in the face. This may be the really difficult point: can a couple accept the inevitable and live with it; or if they cannot accept it, what do they do further?

Grieving for fertility

That infertility is a major loss like others described in this book is not in question. But whereas a visible loss is something to which the couple themselves and their friends and relations can relate to, infertility is a loss of a dream, hope, or an image. A woman may, and probably will, feel that she is not a real woman. She will feel unfulfilled in her very essence of womanhood. And a man will also feel less than a man and perhaps ashamed that he is not able to establish his manhood in his own eyes and those of the people around him. An infertile couple may feel cheated by fate, unable to give their creativity to the world as they had been led to believe and expect.

Just as bereaved spouses may go through a time when they hate any couple they see, so infertile couples may be made aware of their disappointment and inability every time they see a pram or a small baby. Grieving for what one has not is therefore as difficult as grieving for what one has had.

Women who have been thrust into premature menopause because of surgical or hormonal interventions may feel this sense of loss particularly acutely.

The sense of emptiness and uselessness of the body can be quite overwhelming. The reproductive organs are visible and probably functioning outwardly in perfect order, but something uncontrollable is nevertheless going on. In the next chapter health will be considered as a loss also, but here it is not health as such which has been 'lost', rather than a kind of health which has never been there. When we think of 'loss' we think of something which we had in terms of additions to our own life, such as a spouse, a house or a career. In infertility the couple mourns for something which is intrinsic to their bodies. This very fact may also mean that a couple mourn by themselves, not perhaps able to share with others their grief, loss and feelings. Sharing would be even more admitting their helplessness and unfulfilment as persons. So by putting on a brave face, a couple may deny their deepest feelings. This was clearly the case in the story of Heather and James.

The help which such a couple – or the individual in a couple – may need above all is to be shown unconditional positive regard. This will be the aspect of counselling particularly considered in this chapter.

Unconditional positive regard

The *core conditions* which Carl Rogers, the 'founding father' of counselling, said should be present in every helping relationship, are genuineness, warmth and empathy (Rogers, 1980, p. 116). 'Rogers argued that the relationship that develops between counsellor and client is the most significant agent for change, not the counsellor's repertoire of techniques' (Bayne *et al.*, 1994, p. 31). Because of this emphasis on the relationship, Rogers also maintained that these core conditions were both necessary and sufficient. Most forms of counselling, however, also regard them as important, though perhaps not exclusively so. Because of their importance, and because of the different emphasis placed on them, the actual words used and the order in which they are placed vary in the different schools and models. Without going into the details here of such theories, the core conditions will be referred to by different words at times. Indeed, Rogers himself uses 'warmth' and 'unconditional positive regard' interchangeably.

The main concern here is the climate needed for the helping relationship to flourish. This is clearly important in a long-term counselling relationship, but in short and one-off interactions it is also necessary. It is only in a climate of positive acceptance that change can happen. As helpers we have to be constantly aware that we cannot change others; we can help others to change themselves. We cannot tell them in which way they should change; we can, with care, help them to see the world around them in a more realistic light. We can help others to see their feelings, memories and fears in perspective; we cannot tell them in which way they should be feeling and remembering. For this work, then, as helpers we need to be 'experiencing a positive, acceptant attitude toward whatever the client *is* at that moment' (Rogers, 1980, p. 116). When a helper is ready to let a person 'to hang out' whatever is going on at the time: fear, anger, guilt, resentment, pride, fantasies, confusion, then that person is not afraid to mention all this. The atmosphere is one of warmth and aceptance. This is the basis for possible change.

When the helpers and counsellors are 'warm', the client can also be 'warm', that is, when there is unconditional positive regard from the helper to the client, then the client can also be unconditionally positive with himself or herself, and share this with the helper. The relationship which thus develops becomes the main vehicle for the change needed.

Having unconditional positive regard does not mean having no views on anything and being naive. But the starting point is a commitment to the person, not to the problem. This allows for the person herself or himself to come to those 'personal resources they need for positive personality change' (Bayne *et al.*, 1994, p. 31), and when this is addressed and acknowledged with a non-judgemental attitude, there is no need to judge and correct anyway. Thus the helper first of all respects the person. Egan (1990, p. 66) quotes Rogers (1967, p. 102) elaborating unconditional positive regard as meaning that 'the therapist communicates to his client a deep and genuine caring for him as a person with potentialities, a caring uncontaminated by evaluations of his thoughts, feelings or behaviors'. Today we would perhaps say that we see a person in a holistic, rather than in a conditional way.

'Warmth' does not necessarily mean effusiveness. Some people can be very warm without any obvious and external signs. By being with the other person in such a way that both know that this time is theirs, that both are 'engaged' with each other, means being non-possessive. When we can also convey a sense of 'being with' quite unconditionally, that is, there is no hurry, no *need* to achieve, no precondition, then the possibility is great that in fact something *will* be achieved and changed. It is simply not determined beforehand.

The other core conditions (genuineness and empathy) will be considered in the next two chapters.

Other helper attitudes

The one thing which infertility brings with it is a great sense of hope: that everything will work out in the end, even if it is achieved with great personal sacrifice. This may mean, as Speck (1978, p. 43) points out, that the grief process may be delayed because there is also the hope that a new drug or technique may be available to help the couple to conceive and bear a child. Helping an infertile couple may therefore be quite difficult as they may fluctuate emotionally between grieving and hoping, never knowing which is more real or more important.

The attitudes which we bring to a helping relationship are personal attributes which convey that we want to be with *this* person *now*. Such attitudes are of prime importance. It is not possible to say that a person is counselling when in fact what is happening is that the world is being put to rights.

A non-judgemental attitude is necessary if we are to hear what a person is saying, or trying to say. When we are not attending entirely to the other person, we hear only our own thoughts, answers and assumptions. It is remarkable how often this does in fact happen. Most of us are quick to finish another person's sentence, put words into mouths, reach con-clusions and generally believe that everybody holds the same views and values as we do. Perhaps the worst 'sin' in this line is 'I know exactly how you feel'. We do not have to *know* how a person feels from our own experience: we have to hear that person himself or herself saying how he or she feels.

This can be particularly difficult for nurses and health care personnel generally who are active people who like to do things and solve problems. It may therefore take not just a change of gear to switch into the listening mode, but it may actually take a conscious effort to learn how to listen.

Some of the other attitudes which are needed for helping generally, and for helping people with their losses and bereavements in particular, are giving attention, being hopeful and being supportive.

Giving attention

The story of Heather and James shows how the attention of Denise, the practice nurse, helped to bring material to the surface which was needing to be brought up, but which other-wise might have stayed hidden for a very long time yet, per-haps gradually eroding Heather's self-confidence as a person and possibly also her marriage. Denise paid attention to Hea-ther's body language more than anything else in this story. Denise noticed the drawn looks and the restlessness and paid attention to them. With attention we 'tend' towards the per-son, not only physically, but also metaphorically. We become 'all ears'. We have all experienced such listening and being listened to, perhaps in settings which may be quite unlikely, forgetting the surroundings. Who has not met a friend in a supermarket or a station, realizing an hour later that the world had gone on around them but they had not been aware of it? Clearly this is not possible every time we are with another person, but when it does happen, we know we have been in a privileged place.

Giving attention gives a person the permission to be honest. From this point of view, giving attention is not prying or pushing. When there is attention, there is a much greater likelihood of both persons being honest and saying 'no' or 'yes' to the invitation to talk, and meaning it. In the story, Heather first hesitated, and Denise respected this, but also gave her more chances later to talk.

This way of attending shows also the qualities needed by those who use counselling skills, as opposed to those who do counselling. Denise needed to be aware of Heather and respond to her at the time given and in the manner possible. When there is no contract, the timing and manner of helping need to be very fine-tuned. This is not nearly so pronounced in counselling, where two people meet at a fixed time and for a known purpose. When using counselling skills there is spontaneous helping based on spontaneous contact and needs.

Being hopeful

Helping another person would not be possible if the helper did not have some kind of unshakeable belief in the future and in the fact that people can and do change. People who have been bereaved are often stuck at certain emotional points where the impact of the shock experienced may have hit hardest. Being in such a state is depressing enough and when other demands come on top of this, it is sometimes easiest to stay with 'the devil one knows' and refuse to move on. This is a natural enough reaction, but when it becomes a permanent state, it becomes pathological. But telling someone to get on with it, pull themselves together, or see sense is judgemental, showing more our own needs than those of the person concerned. We need to hear the other, but we also need to believe – and convey this belief – that something better is possible. The twelfth century English mystic Julian of Norwich used the phrase 'all will be well, and all will be well, and all manner of thing will be well'. This is surely not just an optimistic ditty, but a guide to the kind of hope which

has the power to overcome present problems, however great
and bleak they may be.

With an attitude of attentiveness, respecting the person
with whom we are, we show this basic hope already. We convey to the person that she or he is worth it; that we are not
thinking we are wasting time; that we are genuine with our
thoughts, words and deeds.

Being supportive

The last of the helper attitudes considered here is that of
being supportive. As everyone who has ever been involved
with a bereaved person knows, ongoing support is one of the
essentials needed for adjustment and resolution. Because
bereavement is different for every person, committing oneself
to support a bereaved person may be a long and sometimes
difficult task. Many bereaved people have experienced that
people around them get impatient very quickly if they are not
over the worst in a fortnight, or over 'it' altogether in six
months. Not only is this unrealistic, it is also insensitive.
There will always be losses to which we can adjust in a short
space of time, but even these will bring with them their memories and significant dates when new aspects might emerge
again.

Being supportive can take many different forms. At one
level detailing the various helper attitudes here is simply considering different facets of the core condition of unconditional
positive regard, and many other words could be added to the
list of such attitudes. In different situations, different aspects
of attitudes may also be more significant, and readers may
easily find words to express what they may need at different times.

Being supportive means above all conveying that we do not
give up. A bereaved person may go through many ups and
downs, and particularly in the stage of developing awareness
(Speck, 1978) or ambivalence (Kübler-Ross, 1969) there may
be times when the person feels very well and says that she
or he feels better, and then for no apparent reason that person
may be in the depths of despair within minutes. Being supportive in such an instance means accepting what is happening, not criticizing and not losing heart that all the good
work done so far is now lost.

If a helper is to be supportive, that helper has to have some
understanding of the process of bereavement and the impli-

cations of loss on a person. But since we all experience these things, it may need little more than common sense to be able to have empathy. What it does take is the courage to be with another person. It may not take a long time, but the quality of that 'being' with another is crucial.

Other helper skills

Helper attitudes are the necessary preconditions for creating a good relationship, but the rest of the helping repertoire is also needed. This consists of the skills of counselling and the skills of relating in general. Some model of helping, such as the Four Questions Model outlined earlier, is also helpful.

With attitudes like unconditional positive regard, being attentive, helpful and supportive, the scene is set for the first question, 'what is happening?' The physical and emotional stance of the helper gives the message 'tell me more; I want to hear what you have to say'. This is not a curious enquiry, but a genuine offer to hear what the person has to say. Most of us know that when we are given the chance to say our piece, the telling of the story itself is therapeutic. We understand something when we hear ourselves say it. When we speak, we do it usually in company, and this means that we get a response from the other person. This in turn stimulates our thinking and understanding. The same is not true when we sit and think by ourselves. Being given the chance to think aloud is therefore a gift which is very precious. But helping is more than just passing the time of day. It is *helping*, that is, this listening is done with a purpose. The listening which is attentive, conveying hope and support, is a directed kind of listening. The patient or client and the helper may not know the direction at all to begin with, but in the talking the direction (the goal) emerges, and this is the core of helping.

The skills of listening, reflecting and challenging (see Chapters 9–12) are clearly also needed. It is such basic skills which turn any relationship into a helping one.

It is very likely that nurses and health professionals meet clients and patients in the course of their work who can be said to be mourning because of their present state of ill health, or because some present problem has triggered an older and perhaps unresolved grief. Such people may not fit neatly into any stages of bereavement or adjustment. Therefore the initial listening may have to be more careful and acute than usual so that the helper may get some idea of what is happening.

The story of Heather highlights also the point that sometimes clients may feel that they are betraying a partner or friend by talking about a difficulty. Heather clearly felt guilty about mentioning the injunction put upon her by her husband. She may also feel uncomfortable admitting that she has gone along with this, for fear of being labelled weak or not assertive. When it is possible for helpers in such situations to show that they are not in any way judging their clients, they will have gained the trust of their clients. It may then be very helpful to acknowledge that they realize that admitting such things may not have been easy. Being supportive may show itself in such ways.

The various attitudes, skills and models are necessary at every stage of grieving and of helping. It can be helpful to bear in mind the four tasks of mourning described by Worden (1991, pp. 10–18): to accept the reality of the loss; to work through to the pain of grief; to adjust to an environment in which the deceased is missing; to emotionally relocate the deceased and move on with life, when meeting someone in need of help with a bereavement. What can sometimes be particularly helpful is actually telling a person that he or she is going through a bereavement when this word may not have been applied to what they are experiencing, as was noted by the person above, whose nurse told her that she was grieving after a miscarriage. In our compartmentalized way of thinking we often do not equate one form of experience with another because we see them as different. Perhaps the most important thing which we can do is to concentrate on the *person*, not the problem, and when we do that, we can make connections, see wholes, relate past and present – all because we give unconditional positive regard to someone who may have been severely damaged by life.

Further reading

Houghton, D. and Houghton, P. (1987) *Coping with Childlessness*. London: Unwin.

Mack, S. and Tucker, J. (1996) *Fertility Counselling*. London: Baillière Tindall.

Mason, M-C. (1993) *Male Infertility — Men Talking*. London: Routledge.

Morley, B. (1996) Grieving for what has never been. *Contact; The Interdisciplinary Journal of Pastoral Studies*, **120**, pp. 22–25.

Pfeffer, N. & Woolett, A.N. (1983) *The Experience of Infertility*. London: Virago.

Read, J. (1995) *Counselling for Fertility Problems*. London: Sage.

CHAPTER SEVEN

Loss of health
Congruence
....

Gareth was in hospital for a series of investigations. He had not been feeling well lately, and his GP had referred him to the local genito-urinary clinic. Gareth was not very happy there and protested that he was in the wrong place. So he came to talk to a student nurse.

Gareth was 62, but looked more like 42. Five years ago his partner, Philip, had died. Gareth could never accept that he had died of kidney failure. Philip had been on the waiting list for a kidney transplant, but he died before an organ became available. Gareth blamed himself for not doing enough to get a kidney.

When Philip was first investigated, about ten years ago, both of them had HIV tests, and Gareth tested positive, but Philip was negative. Gareth was immediately dismissed from his job as school caretaker. He never managed to find another job. He spent his life helping other people as much as he could. When therefore his partner became seriously ill, he looked after him. When Philip died, Gareth became depressed and began to wonder why it was not he who had died. But in fact he was actually physically well. He had another test, and this one turned out negative. It then transpired that the first test had been wrongly positive. Gareth had lost his job and livelihood unjustly. He started compensation proceedings. This needed a psychiatric assessment. Because of his depression, Gareth often talked of wanting to die; this jeopardized his chances for getting the compensation.

His own hurt at the wrong result, his guilt over not having helped his partner more and his wish to die now made him conscious of every pain and malfunction of his body, and his mistrust of tests and medical personnel simply compounded the situation.

Rosemary was 38. She had had a second baby only three months earlier and was still breastfeeding him when one day she discovered a lump in her left breast. This was quickly diagnosed as malignant. She had to wean her baby and get on with surgery and treatments. As she was going to the hospital one day for her radiotherapy, she *fell on an uneven pavement and broke her right arm. This was hard, having to have her arm in plaster and trying still to look after a small baby. She made a good recovery, but after two years she showed signs of bony metastases. She had more radiotherapy. Then she had hypercalcaemia, and had more treatment. In the meantime her mother had a stroke and died two weeks later. Her first child was involved in a minor accident and also had to have hospital treatment, thankfully not for long.*

Rosemary tried every suggestion for helping her to get better, but she realized that she was losing the battle against cancer. She often had pain and needed to rest. Her liver became enlarged and caused breathlessness.

The sense of paying for the life of her second child with her own life was often acute. She wondered if all this would not have happened if she had not had another child; she had wanted this child very much. Could her husband manage? What will the children do without their mother? Many thoughts went through her mind. She would often talk with the night nurses when she was in hospital having treatments of one kind or another.

About six months before she died, she had gone through a particularly dark moment emotionally. It felt as if she was asked gradually to give everything back she had received during her life. She and her husband often talked about this, too. From somewhere, she knew not quite where, the thought came to ask her husband to marry again. Alison, her sister, had always been close to all of them, and had been helping them while Rosemary was ill. They discussed the possibility of Alison marrying her husband. Rosemary felt it would be easier to die, knowing this possibility existed. She had given back even her own marriage.

Losing one's health

Perhaps the paradoxes of birth and death and health and illness are best captured in poetry. Dylan Thomas (1914–1953) had a way of saying the unsayable:

Oh isn't life a terrible thing, thank God?

(*Under Milk Wood*, 1954)

We can lose our health in accidents and within moments, but that, on the whole, is temporary. Or we can lose our health through disease and illness, and that often means gradually, but relentlessly. And there is the loss of mental health, which can be insidious and painful, but with the body functioning normally.

There are also many other forms of 'loss' of health, such as physical handicaps present from birth, chronic diseases, like diabetes, which are not usually debilitating when controlled.

It is also nearly impossible to say that someone is completely healthy. Being healthy is an experience more than a measurable fact. In the same way, some people can be visibly or measurably unhealthy, but not experience themselves as ill.

Short-term loss of health

All of us experience times of incapacitation due to colds, migraines and other minor illnesses. We do not consider these to be significant experiences generally, and rightly so. Life is made up of a constant quest to keep illness and health in balance and most of us have learned to do this reasonably well most of the time.

Losing one's health in an accident or in some other dramatic way, however, can be devastating. We are not prepared for such an onslaught when the whole of life is disrupted. Morse and Carter (1995) describe how a patient, Joan, who had survived an accident in which she was burned and three of her children died, preserved her sense of self. They describe how people in traumatic events 'instinctively find the capacity to survive immense physical and psychological assault'.

Initially Joan was enduring to survive. Then, when she became more physically stable, she was enduring to live. Only when she had reached a point of awareness of her predicament did the suffering begin.

Fortunately only few people have to go through such traumatic events, but the process of

enduring to survive
enduring to live
suffering

is very recognizable by anyone who has been through some form of accident. It is only when these stages have been lived through that some form of adjustment can take place. These stages, described here from the experience of trauma, are very similar to the process of grieving outlined in Chapter 2.

For many people such a traumatic event will divide life into before and after the accident. The accident becomes the point of reference. This may be so even for what may be considered as a 'minor' event, such as breaking an arm or a leg. The circumstances of the event will inevitably contribute to such a sense of division. It is not only the physical pain experienced from an accident, but most of all the disruption and rapid change of environment and life-style which make such events memorable. Even years later, some people remember the exact details of such events.

The impact on families and friends of an accident or traumatic event cannot be overlooked. Depending on the circumstances, they may be as shocked as the person concerned, and their lives may be as much, if not more, disrupted as the actual patient's. Patton (1995), a professor of nursing, describes her experience as a mother to cope with the diagnosis and treatment of cancer of her son David. The event changed her whole life:

I have changed both professionally and personally. ... I have learned about myself, my son, and my relationship with family, friends, and God. ... I will be more sensitive to patient and family questions. ... I will be more aware of the conflicts that others may experience, which may be much like my professional and personal conflict. ... I am not the same person, nor do I want to be. My priorities, both professional and personal, are different. I try to take one day at a time, but it is not always easy. I am coming to grips with the reality that the guarantees I wanted, and still want, do not exist.

Even when health is restored again after a time of illness, there may nevertheless be effects which remain with the person for the rest of life. A scar, pain, diminished function of a limb, or reduced sight or hearing may be constant reminders of the traumatic event. This may contribute to reduced mental health and changes in personality and social contacts. Thus the short-term loss of health can become a chronic one, perhaps slowly and imperceptibly. The changes in the significant people around the patient may be just as great and just as lasting.

Long-term loss of health

The change from an illness which can be cured to one which cannot, may be imperceptible. In the early stages of any illness there is a strong hope that treatments will be successful. Patients have emotional energy to fight whatever illness or disease is present. There may be some form of denial going on, but there may also be a real sense of hope, based on earlier experiences of illness and disease. Depending on the information given and how this can be processed, there should indeed be hope.

Parkes (1975b) describes what happens when patients are given a diagnosis of cancer of the ear, nose and throat:

If the change [in health] is relatively sudden or it has not been expected, the most immediate reaction is likely to be one of numbness and disbelief. 'I just can't take it in. It can't be true'. If the situation is ambiguous, as it usually is in the early stages of cancer, then it may be possible to avoid confronting the reality of what is happening for a considerable length of time, the patient will overlook evidence that his physical state is worsening. Eventually the evidence of deterioration becomes too obvious to ignore and he will then enter a phase of restless anxiety and pining. Having recognized that there is a major discrepancy between the world that is and the world that has been taken for granted up to now, the individual tries every way to get back the world he has lost (emphasis added).

Parkes goes on to describe the other stages of dying outlined by Kübler-Ross (1969), describing anger and aggression, bargaining, depression and acceptance. He describes a patient of his who maintained that 'cancer is all psychological' and believed that God had cured him because he had prayed hard enough. When patients with him in a group planned to visit Lourdes, they discussed miracles of cure and miracles of acceptance. This patient, finding that his cancer had not disappeared, then decided that he had experienced the miracle of acceptance. This is surely not an isolated example, but shows the various means we have of adjusting to disease and loss of health.

The experiences of loss of health take as many different forms as there are people. Hull (1990, p. 47), who is a university professor, describes his gradual loss of sight in his autobiography, and also how he fights his depression.

Occasionally I feel depressed, and this is worst when I am frustrated in playing with the children. I feel as if I have become nothing, unable to act as a father, impotent, unable to survey, to admire, or to exercise jurisdiction or discrimination. I have a strange feeling of being dead. My response is to go even further inwards, into a deeper deadness. I sink into quietness and passivity. I might sit in a chair alone, without moving, reducing my breathing to the barest minimum, simmering down until I am aware of less and less. I try to think of nothing, and often drift in and out of sleep. I might cover myself with a blanket, cutting out any faint sounds, and by emptying myself

completely, I become the cipher that my blindness tells me I am. In this state, I can continue for hours.
This technique for fighting depression is effective up to a point, It does provide a certain refuge, a kind of solace, a place to go.

Coping with long-term illness has many aspects. Using a walking stick, wearing a cervical collar, or having a visible condition makes most people very conscious of not being 'normal' when they are in company. Routine tasks become major procedures. An advert of the Arthritis and Rheumatism Council in 1996 in the British press had a photo of a pair of very crippled hands laid on a surface, with a wrapped sweet between them, with the heading 'For some people a sweet can become a task beyond endurance'. Some people have no visible disability, but a cancer growing inside, of which they are very conscious. Health care workers may get used to seeing people looking grey and drawn and emaciated, but seeing people in the street looking very ill can be a shock. The people themselves may not be aware of their looks, but they are surely aware of how they feel. Sometimes keeping illness from others is as important as sharing it.

Schaefer (1995) describes many losses which women experience in chronic illness: loss of health, support, control, function, spontaneity, truth and perspective. Although Schaefer writes about women, men will certainly experience similar losses. Indeed, she says that women felt that men did not take them seriously: women often say that men are 'soft' and cannot bear pain. The problem is one of not being taken seriously. No-one has time to listen to people's detailed problems. In a society where we expect more and more that there is an answer to very problem and a pill for every ill, having a condition or disease which cannot be cured is somehow unacceptable. The sufferers therefore blame themselves. When the illness has anything to do with the sexual and reproductive organs, there may be a sense of shame and guilt. Denying what the illness is or is about can then be a way of coping with it. But when an illness has to be kept from others, there is another sense of loss present: that of being honest with oneself and with others. The sense of being alone and having to turn inwards for either comfort or oblivion can become isolating.

Sometimes it is not loss of total health which is the problem, but some aspect of health. Facial disfigurement has been well documented (e.g. Rhŷs-Evans, 1996), and so has also the loss of a breast or a limb. A laryngectomy (Weber and Reimer,

1993) can mean that a person is disfigured and has problems with speech and fluid production, but can otherwise be well for years. Without much help such a person may be very self-conscious in company and become unnecessarily reclusive.

Mental illness is such a vast subject that it can at best only be acknowledged here. Sometimes it is claimed that every person suffers from some kind of mental illness at some stage in life. But the relatively short periods of depression which most people know can hardly be called 'illness' as such, since they do little more than make life somewhat more difficult for a time. The recognized forms of mental illness, such as mania, pathological depression and schizophrenia, often mark people for life and they need years of treatment of some form or another.

The mental illnesses which occur in later life, such as Alzheimer's Disease and other dementias, often mean that the person is not really aware of the condition, unlike mental illnesses in younger persons. The loss of identity (Orona, 1990) which occurs in these types of illnesses is usually more distressing for the family and carers of the persons concerned than for the sufferers themselves. This can mean that not one life is disrupted – and therefore grieved for – but several. The dynamics which result from this can be far-reaching.

People who have had strokes sometimes find themselves in peculiar situations where they may dissociate themselves from the paralysed parts. Speck (1978, p. 105) writes of a woman who remarked

I lay in bed thinking, 'Why am I dead on one side? Is this what death is like, dying in little bits? I know what I'm saying but why doesn't anyone understand me?' I was not sure at that time whether I would live or die and when people did not seem to respond to my words, although I thought I was talking clearly, I wondered if I was already dead. I was very frightened.

The loss of health is a kind of death. Very often it is also the first step on the road to death. This is why illness is inevitably feared. With the loss of health goes a loss of personhood and a shattering of dreams and hopes. But loss is not all there is to it. The way in which people respond and react to illness and loss of health shows their true personality. The 'ideal' might be that someone accepts the loss and so becomes peaceful in the face of impending death. Some people also find new energy – perhaps born of anger – on being given a diagnosis of cancer. Yet others use a disability not only to their own advantage, but also to that of often countless other people.

Congruence

The aim of helping those who are bereaved of a person, of health, or of an ideal, is not so much to help them get 'over' it as to get *through* it.

The shock of the event will have caused a kind of wall to be erected between the bereaved and the world. This is a protective wall, but in time it can also become a wall of separation between reality and the self and between other people and the self. Worden (1991, p. 16) says that people who do not carry out Task III of his model (To adjust to an environment in which the deceased is missing), promote their own helplessness, do not develop the skills they need to cope, withdraw from the world and do not face up to the environmental requirements. The wall which they therefore maintain around themselves has first to be recognized, then acknowledged, and then dealt with.

There are several ways of dealing with walls:

One can bang one's head against it, ending up with a big headache at best, or a cracked skull at worst
One can leap over it
One can dig under it (as Hull, 1990, described it)
One can take it down
One can try to find the door in it
One can make a door in it.

The task of helping and counselling is to give the client an opportunity to see and perhaps try each of these possible ways of dealing with a problem. Perhaps the most productive way may be for the client to learn how to take the wall down himself or herself, or to find the door which exists. In this metaphorical way of describing a problem, it is possible that if a wall is jumped, that one can jump back again. Going through the door has a sense of being able also to lock it, once through, and to give the key away or bury it.

When considering the second of the core conditions for successful helping, congruence, it is important to remember that both people in the relationship have to be congruent. But the helper has the professional responsibility of creating the atmosphere in which helping can take place. The helper consciously contributes this. This is so if it is a therapeutic relationship with a contract, or a short, one-off occasion when counselling skills are used. We can only help if we are also prepared to lead in the only real way possible.

The words congruence, genuineness, or realness have all been used interchangeably to mean a certain transparency (Rogers, 1980, p. 115):

the therapist makes himself or herself transparent to the client; the client can see right through what the therapist is in the relationship; the client experiences no holding back on the part of the therapist. As for the therapist, what he or she is experiencing is available to aware-ness, can be lived in the relationship, and can be communicated, if appropriate. Thus there is a close matching, or congruence, between what is being experienced at the gut level, what is present in aware-ness, and what is expressed to the client.

This is a tall order and can sound impossible. In my own experience it takes perhaps years for a helper or counsellor to come to this kind of transparency. It takes much experience to be able to be completely honest with oneself and convey this in such a manner as to also help the client. When it does happen – perhaps only at one or two points in an interaction – both people in the relationship know that something important has happened. The fact that this congruence is dif-ficult to achieve and may be an ideal more than reality, does not make it any the less important; on the contrary, it is some-thing which helpers should strive for constantly.

Being congruent can mean something like the following. A nurse is with a patient who is trying to become stabilized on insulin. The patient gets frustrated and does not want to hear any more what the nurse is saying. The nurse realizes that this may be due to a sense of grieving going on for the patient, in which she adjusts to the diabetes and the new status of a chronically sick person. The nurse says that he understands and that they can go over the procedure again. This nurse has made allowances for the patient's feelings, but not for his own. He may feel just as frustrated as the patient: at her for not wanting to learn, and at himself for not getting through to her. But he keeps his own feelings to himself, goes away and per-haps 'blows his top' to a colleague, blaming the patient. He is not congruent in that he does not acknowledge his feelings, and by telling the patient he understands, but telling a col-league that he is fed up with the patient, he is not congruent.

On the other hand, if the nurse tells the patient there and then that he is frustrated, this does not help either of them. Both feel helpless because both are thus paralysed by their inabilities to achieve a goal.

The nurse would be congruent if he told the patient something like:

I can see that you are getting frustrated, and I can well understand you. I am also getting frustrated because I am not helping you well enough. In this way we are disabling each other. Let's take a moment to see what we could do to help each other.

Neither hiding feelings nor blurting them out is helpful. But being aware of feelings, and considering carefully how much to share with the client at this moment and how much to share later or elsewhere, is a skill which helps. Clients are as smart as helpers in reading body language, and when helpers try to suppress some strong feelings, either of anger, frustration or love, clients notice this just as surely as we do. Trying to hide or deny what is going on may then damage the relationship. Knowing something about the dynamics of relationships, in particular helping relationships, is therefore essential. But just as necessary is being versed in communication and helping skills. We cannot be versed only in one aspect of helping; all the aspects go together.

How to help people who suffer loss of health

All the authors of books providing guidance for counsellors (e.g. Worden, 1991; Raphael, 1984; Rando, 1984), and those whose articles have been cited throughout this book, give some indication on how best to help. This is the reason for establishing models and processes. And yet, when it comes to actually being with a person, most of us feel as if on virgin ground, having to learn on the spot, think on one's feet, and perhaps even deliberately forget theories because we are with a real, live person. Every situation calls for a unique approach. This is not a drawback, but the real challenge of helping. It is also what makes helping and counselling both so attractive and so demanding.

Helping Gareth

When considering congruence in particular in relation to the story of Gareth, there is one outstanding factor. Gareth wanted to be ill so that he could die, and he also wanted to get the compensation and this meant needing to show that he wanted to live. He therefore gave conflicting messages. This could be quite difficult enough for an experienced counsellor, let alone for a student nurse. Perhaps just because Gareth mistrusted doctors and tests, which is understandable given his history, he might have chosen to talk to a student who might not (yet) know too much. It is likely that the student nurse picks up very soon that Gareth does not really know what he wants, to die or to live. All health care workers are oriented towards helping and getting better, especially in someone who looks so apparently healthy and young like Gareth. The conflict produced in the student nurse may therefore be quite considerable. Can he really help Gareth? Should he even attempt to help? The student nurse can ask himself these question, and he can ask Gareth, too. They are the basic questions 'what is happening?' and 'what is the meaning of it?' in a different form. If the student nurse is concentrating only on his feelings, then he will soon be exasperated. If he shows this to Gareth in any kind of way, they end up talking at each other rather than with each other. If the student nurse admits that he is not sure where he is, what is wanted of him, how he can help, then he may actually be doing the best thing in the way of help: being congruent. In this way Gareth has to say what he wants and needs. This may not be what is actually best for him in the long-term view of a goal, but what he will probably need in the short term is being listened to and taken seriously. He has been dismissed too often in the past: given a wrong diagnosis, dismissed from his job because of it, 'dismissed' by his partner, dismissed by the GP to another doctor. If, with congruence, the student nurse finds that what Gareth wants and needs is unconditional positive regard – not being dismissed here – then he is helping him in the best way possible. Being listened to may be the first thing which he needs very badly. It may be that the student nurse is able to help him to see that in fact he is grieving not just for his partner, but also for his health, destroyed some ten years ago, on paper, but in a very real sense for him also, by robbing him of a livelihood. Acknowledging such facts may help Gareth to begin to make sense of a difficult position, and perhaps help him to look for a door in the wall which he had built around himself and against which he now constantly banged his head, giving him (metaphorically) a very sore head.

It is usually easier to help a person who is attractive and is also willing to do her or his bit in the process of adjusting and changing to new circumstances. It does not mean that we cannot help the unfriendly or the unattractive. But we cannot help the unwilling. We cannot change others; we can only change ourselves. If therefore we feel cold and angry towards some persons, this should be acknowledged, but not to their face. It is not their 'fault' that *we* feel like that. Being aware of the feelings may help *us* to realize that *we* need help.

We cannot make a person to change and see the error of his or her ways. We can acknowledge that someone should change, and offer help, but we should always be aware that this offer can be rejected. However, with sensitive help, it may be possible for a person to come to some insights and change.

Helping Rosemary

All the other aspects of helping discussed in this book also come into force when helping Rosemary with the loss of her health. If she looks for help from the nursing staff – or from other helpers available – the fact that she is mourning her loss of health is the starting point. When looking at her story from the point of view of congruence, some of the following observations apply also.

Whereas it may be quite difficult for nurses to empathize with Gareth, just the opposite may happen with Rosemary. She has gone through a great deal of suffering, and the way she expresses this suffering to people may mean that people can identify with her and perhaps feel sorrow with and for her. This sort of thing should not happen to her – the world is a cruel and unjust place. Maybe there is something in her story which also touches our own story, making it easier to relate to her.

The warmth mentioned in the last chapter could mean that, faced with a person like Rosemary, a nurse might want to throw her arms around her and feel sorry for her. Or empathy, which will be discussed in the next chapter, may be understood to be walking in her shoes. How then is one congruent in such situations? Is a nurse congruent when she or he feels very warm towards Rosemary in this room, and quite the opposite to Gareth in the next room?

Clearly we do not feel the same for and with every person, and rightly so. Congruence here means first of all acknowledging our own feelings for and to another person. Being aware of how we feel in a situation does not mean that these feelings are necessarily the right ones or that everybody will feel the same. It means that we acknowledge that we cannot understand this man; feel protective towards this woman; are aware of frustration here, or feel real love for someone now and would like to express this. Being aware of our feelings, emotions and sensations can mean that we can use these aspects of ourselves when helping another person. We may be able to share with the other person how we feel now, or say that this is uppermost in the mind. Perhaps the other person is experiencing similar feelings at the same time? It may be that our feelings and emotions are blocking our capacity to listen. We become aware of ourselves and thus unable to be aware of the other person and what is happening to him or her. Simply stating what is happening may then unblock the free flow of attention. When this is done, it does usually not mean that the conversation is disrupted; on the contrary, it may mean that the flow is restored again by giving attention to what is happening now. Congruence is only valid when it is seen in the context of the other core conditions, and of the counselling skills needed for a successful relationship.

Further reading   Clubb, R.L. (1991) Chronic sorrow: adaptation patterns of parents with chronically ill children. *Pediatric Nursing* **17** (5): 461–466.

Faulkner, A. and Maguire, P. (1994) *Talking to Cancer Patients and Their Relatives*. Oxford: Oxford University Press.

Frayley, A.M. (1990) Chronic sorrow: a parental response. *Journal of Pediatric Nursing* **5** (4): 268–273.

Hales, G. (1995) *Beyond Disability: Towards an Enabling Society*. Milton Keynes: Open University.

Hull, J.M. (1990) *Touching the Rock*. London: Arrow Books.

Karp, D.A. (1996) *Speaking of Sadness; Depression, Disconnection and the Meanings of Illness*. New York: Oxford University Press.

Larson, D.G. (1993) *The Helper's Journey: Working With People Facing Grief, Loss and Life-threatening Illness*. Champaign, IL: Research.

Lyons, R., Sullican, M.J.L., Ritvo, P.G., Coyne, J.C. (1995) *Relationships in Chronic Illness and Disability*. London: Sage.

CHAPTER EIGHT

Divorce and separation
Empathy

....

Angus was furious when he found a photo of Roland, their neighbour, in Sally's handbag. He had begun to be suspicious a few weeks ago that something was going on, and with the chance to look through her handbag, he had his evidence. He did not conceal his fury when Sally came in from collecting the children from school.

Angus and Sally had been married for nearly 20 years. Their children, now aged ten and twelve, were conceived by artificial insemination because Angus suffered from multiple sclerosis. This had started some months before their wedding, but had not been diagnosed by the time they got married. They were a happy couple, on the whole, and had a good family life. Angus was disabled to some degree, but during times of remission coped well. Because he had to have treatments on a more or less regular basis, he was well known to the local GP and her team, including the health visitor, Cathy.

When the 'discovery' was made, events moved fast. Sally had already planned to move out of the house, leaving Angus and the children in their home. Not unexpectedly, Angus had a relapse of his MS, and Cathy heard much of the story, trying to help Angus. He had an enormous need to talk.

Although Sally moved out, she had not envisaged a divorce, but Angus had no doubt. If a mother would not look after her children, then she was not fit to remain a wife either. He started divorce proceedings as soon as he could.

Sheila and Robert had been married about two years. Sheila was a successful dress designer, full of energy and ideas. Robert was a musician with a promising career. They were both strong personalities, both of them coming from families with dominant mothers. Sheila's family were also 'well-to-do' and there were all the necessary comforts in their adequately large flat. After about a year of marriage, Robert hit a period when he had little work. He was at home much of the time, content to call himself a 'house-husband'. He had *dinner ready for Sheila most evenings and the flat had never been so clean. Robert was proud and mentioned a few times that the flat should remain in good shape even after he got busy again.*

Sheila met many interesting people at her work, once or twice having to go away for a night on business. On one of these trips she met Carl and had a passionate affair with him. When she told Robert, he felt totally betrayed and they separated a week later. Sheila moved out of her flat, but she knew that Carl would never be the person to share life with: a night or two, yes, but not much more.

Robert and Sheila stayed in touch, over the years having a stormy relationship. When Sheila was in hospital for a hysterectomy, her primary nurse told her that she was separating from her husband, and the two women got talking, exchanging experiences. The nurse was struck by how often Sheila mentioned the word 'guilt'. She asked Sheila what this was about, and that was when Sheila told her some of the details. The nurse said to Sheila that she was not a trained counsellor, but perhaps there might be some way of exploring this guilt together. After all, it was also something which she was acquainted with.

Divorce and separation

Divorce is so common these days that when their parents have a dispute, some children already fear that they are going to separate. A divorce or separation is terrible enough for the adults, but the children probably suffer just as much, though differently.

A separation does not usually happen overnight. There is a gradual build-up of tension and an equally gradual loss of the relationship as it once existed. All close relationships change, but for a partner relationship to deteriorate, there needs to be some withdrawal of the commitment once made. If there had not been a commitment in the first place, there would not be the possibility of a separation.

While most of the aspects considered in this book concern losses which make one sad and over which one may have little control, divorce and separation are a choice – not always willed – and can also be a very good thing for some people. But while it may be a liberation for one partner, it may be an agony for the other. One may gain and the other may lose.

The grief which may go with a separation may be compounded because the other partner is still alive and it is always possible that one meets the other again. A divorce is a kind of death with the 'dead' person still living. It can be very embarrassing when ex-partners meet by chance in a public place.

It is not just the couple who divorce; the families which had been created by their coming together now also divorce. Grandchildren may not see their grandparents again, children may not see their cousins again. Complex new families are created, with step-children and half-brothers and sisters. This can be wonderful; it can also be confusing. One parent can become the good parent – usually the one with whom the children spend less time – and the other parent may become the bad one.

Separation often means a fall in income and consequent restrictions for the children. They have nothing against either parent, and therefore they see their separation as very selfish and making them bear pain which has nothing to do with them. They can become resentful and hate a parent. In the case of Angus, he had the custody of the children, and the girl did not want to visit her mother in the home of her new partner. She could not forgive her mother for robbing her of a family and she let her know it by her behaviour.

Whereas for most losses of a person through old age or illness there is little in the way of a search for the cause, in separation there is normally a great deal of searching going on. Why did it happen? Could it have been prevented? Accusations and self-accusations are common. Marriage is an ideal, but to turn this into reality seems to have been beyond the capabilities of the partners.

Marriage was never more popular, never more risky than it is today. The popularity extends to second and third marriages, the risk arises from a combination of high expectations and of tough social pressures. In consequence, breakdown, one-parent families and complicated step-relationships are now part of our normal social fabric. (Thompson, 1987, p. 55)

Dominian (1968) lists a number of reasons why marriages break down, citing among others intelligence, a parental image, dependency, childhood deprivation, and self-esteem. The expectations one has of a marriage vary with every person and every couple. Some marry for love, others for security, some for money and yet others to get away from parents or families. For some people, love at first sight is what they want, and for others this would never do.

Davis and Murch (1992, p. 178) also point out that men and women have different expectations of marriage. Women have become more vocal about demanding what they want, and not simply being there to do the husband's pleasure. They say that 'the "emancipation of women" has ... had an impact on divorce rates in two ways: firstly, in provoking more women to question the terms of the bargain which they appear to have struck, and secondly, in giving them freedom to leave'.

The image of marriage has changed so drastically in the last few decades that it is often difficult for people to know what they might or should look for in a marriage. Parental values may still be very strong, yet combined with what young people see happening around them, these values may clash with what they now actually experience. Most people will have known some elderly relatives who only stayed together because divorce was not an option in their social circles. They may still live together, but more out of habit than love. But a young couple may still want their elderly relatives to accept their very different relationship.

When a relationship begins to show signs of a breakdown, there is often the hope that it can be mended again. Marriage guidance counsellors and mediators are much in demand in our society. Their role is usually one of third party through which the couple can address each other. With another person present, it is often easier to express the inexpressible. The atmosphere in which this is done is neutral, that is, not in the home of either partner. The expectation is also that relationships can heal and work again, and that divorce is not inevitable when the going gets tough.

The loss in divorce

A marriage is normally regarded as the act of committing oneself to the person one has chosen to share one's deepest feelings and longings with, not simply one's goods and possessions. There is a bond which was created between two people when they looked each other in the eye and recognized there their 'other half': that part of themselves which was missing in order to be a complete person. This does not necessarily mean that the other person is supplementing what is not there, but that the other has the capacity to call forth that which is necessary, to come to a greater whole. Not only is there a great expectation that the partner will be the ideal, right and only person with whom to share life, but there is also the expectation that because of that person, we ourselves are the ideal, right and only person for the partner. When this hope and vision does not come true, there is not only a loss of the other person; there is also the loss of a hope, of a belief in the other and in oneself, and a loss of a vision and ideal. There is perhaps for the first time

in life a recognition that we are limited people and less capable than we had imagined. By letting go of such fundamental
values we are letting ourselves down, and also all those who
had supported us in our quest in this marriage. The loss is
therefore perhaps a loss of everything that we stood for and
are. This is a loss indeed. When perhaps on top of this comes
the loss of a home, of a family, income, security and perhaps
a neighbourhood and circle of friends and acquaintances, the
loss can be described as total. No wonder that divorce is often
much more difficult to accept and deal with than the death
of a loved person.

Not unjustly, one partner may feel very resentful. The story
of a decent marriage of 25 years, and then one day the husband walks out, having met a younger woman, may be a Mills
and Boon caricature, but in fact may also be quite close to
reality. The woman will feel that she has given unselfishly to
the marriage, and now she is simply ditched. She may resent
her husband, the years she spent caring for him and the family
and home, perhaps sacrificing a career and other prospects.
She may protest her love, but his mind is made up. Despite
feeling used and useless, she may find it very difficult to
detach herself emotionally from her husband. Perhaps less
common, but just as real, is the story of Angus and Sally. The
love for the departed partner then turns into hate and bitterness. Angus often admitted to getting a 'kick' out of wishing
all manner of ill fortune on his ex-wife and her new partner.
Such feelings are not passing emotions. On the contrary, they
may now give the remaining partner the strength to carry on
living. This is all very well if such feelings turn into positive
forces, but if they remain negative, then it can be said that
the new life is driven by anger, resentment and hate.

The way in which the divorce law operates means that one
partner has to be declared guilty. This means that the other
is seen to be not at fault. Such labelling is often very
important for one or other party, but it means that such labels
also stick. The labels are crude and do not invite either reconciliation or forgiveness. Being judged the 'no fault' party
can be as damaging – emotionally – as being judged the 'guilty' party. In a relationship it is barely possible to say that one
person is entirely at fault and the other is not. It would not
have been a marriage if both people had not interacted.

Empathy

Empathy is not specific to situations of loss from divorce and
separation. Empathy is perhaps the most universally recog-

nized element for helping another person. In order to show what it is and how it can be used, it is specifically applied here to loss from bereavement, of which divorce and separation are part. Empathy applies also in all the other situations discussed in this book.

In the early days of counselling practice, empathy was often seen to be a skill which one could learn and apply. Scales were devised for measuring the amount of empathy shown by a helper. It became evident that one could say something which could be declared as 'empathic', but the client did not perceive it as such. One can say the right words but not show the attitude which goes with the word. Can this still be empathy? Over the years it became evident that empathy could not be measured in the same way as other skills. Empathy, as Rogers (1980) came to demonstrate, is 'a way of being'. First of all, one *is* empathic as a person, only then can one also act empathically. But such statements bring with them all kinds of difficulties. There is not just one way of being empathic. If empathy is a way of being, then there must be as many ways of being empathic as there are people. How can empathy be described and recognized in such circumstances? It is fair to say that Rogers spent much of his later years of life trying to define empathy. In one of his last books (Rogers, 1980, pp. 142–3) he set out his 'current definition', ending it by saying that 'being empathic is a complex, demanding, and strong – yet also a subtle and gentle – way of being'.

(L)et me attempt a description of empathy that would seem satisfactory to me today. I would no longer be terming it a 'state of empathy', because I believe it to be a process, rather than a state. ... It means entering the private perceptual world of the other and becoming thoroughly at home in it. It involves being sensitive, moment by moment, to the changing felt meanings which flow in this other person, to the fear or rage or tenderness or confusion or whatever that he or she is experiencing. It means temporarily living in the other's life, moving about in it delicately without making judgments; it means sensing meanings of which he or she is scarcely aware, but not trying to uncover totally unconscious feelings, since this would be too threatening. It includes communicating your sensings of the person's world as you look with fresh and unfrightened eyes at elements of which he or she is fearful. ... To be with another in this way means that for the time being, you lay aside your own views and values in order to enter another's world without prejudice.

This quotation covers some of the aspects of the helper attitudes described in earlier chapters. It also shows that unconditional positive regard and congruence are part of empathy – and the other way round.

Sometimes empathy is described as 'walking in the other's shoes'. But the quotation makes clear that this is a wrong image. It is not walking in the other's shoes which is called for; that would mean pushing the other out of his or her own shoes – but trying to imagine and understand what it is like for the other to walk in his or her kind of shoes: 'entering the private perceptual world of the other and becoming thoroughly at home in it'. This world may be full of anger, resentment, confusion, grief, fear and lostness. Trying to become at home in it does mean accepting and acknowledging that the other person is feeling these things and that they are real. But 'becoming at home' in them does not mean that we as helpers make these feelings our own. We do not identify with the client to the extent of becoming 'involved with' him or her. We go alongside that person, hear what he or she has to say, and, and in hearing sensitively and being completely 'present' give that person the security of acceptance, from which changes can be made. We cannot make the changes; we can help to provide the climate from within which changes can be made. Such changes may be slow, because the feelings have first to be recognized for what they are, then owned, and only then can they be dealt with appropriately.

The word 'empathy' is often used these days, like 'counselling', without understanding what is actually meant or involved. There is a possibility that it is confused with 'sympathy'. Sympathy means feeling 'with', and can lead to an identification. Two people who have sympathy for each other may be comparing events: a client's situation may remind a helper of a similar event, thus focusing the attention of both people now on that event. This can be confusing for a client who may then find himself or herself in the role of helper. Empathy means feeling 'in', meaning that the helper is able to feel what the other is feeling and acknowledge this, without necessarily bringing in his or her own agenda.

It is not enough that helpers can feel empathy, that is, feel at home in the other's world. This capacity has to be communicated to the other person. This is perhaps what is known as 'accurate empathy' (Egan, 1990, p. 133): sensing accurately what is going on and being able to convey this in such a way that it helps the client to move forward. This is the aim, but clearly we cannot be right or on track or accurate all the time.

Egan points out that in either case, the client usually lets the helper know if a comment or response was accurate. 'Exactly', or 'that's it' are clear enough indications that a remark was right; 'not quite' or 'no, it was more like ...' are indications that this time the helper was off the mark. Normally this sort of interaction does not harm a conversation when it happens occasionally, but if a helper is consistently 'beside the point' then it cannot be called empathy.

Some people are so traumatized that they are not really sure what is going on or what they are feeling. When an empathic helper is able to be accurate in picking up perhaps on just one or two items, or at least on the uppermost ones, then this can sometimes seem like a miracle to a person. 'You read me like a book' can then be a remark which may be a compliment, but what is experienced is a sense of real understanding. This may not seem so incredible to the helper, because he or she has some understanding of the person's predicament. In fact, to be able to lay one's finger on the main problem is just a skill.

Empathic statements are used at any stage of a helping relationship. The question 'what is happening?' invites a person to talk, and in the talking perhaps some order may become apparent. By reflecting (see Chapter 10) some points back to the client, we are empathic. By asking 'what is the meaning of it?' we are asking perhaps the most empathic question. Indeed, it is often not a question which is being asked at this stage, but a statement like 'seeing this clearly has actually given your life a new meaning' is in itself an empathic statement. In this case it is a communication of something heard or sensed from the client.

In any situation of loss and bereavement it is the experience of often unknown, or a confusing array of, feelings which is the difficult part. If we want to help people on an emotional level, as distinct from the practical level – then we need to concentrate on the feelings – or rather on the person-with-the-feelings. Only in this way can we be said to be effective counsellors or persons using counselling skills. By concentrating on the problem, that is, the practical aspects of either disease, illness or affairs of house and job, we do not help a person to change an attitude. When we try to be empathic as helpers, we are more likely to help the person to concentrate on the feelings, emotions and attitudes. Because being empathic involves the skills of listening and reflecting in particular, we help to keep the focus on the person and are less easily distracted. By staying with the feelings through reflection, we consolidate the relationship and the trust which is building up between the two people. This means that more work can be done, now built on a secure foundation of respect and genuineness.

Being empathic with Angus

Cathy, the health visitor, had known Angus for a number of years, and they had always got on well. Cathy visited the house occasionally, particularly when Angus had a relapse and needed more help. It was therefore natural that he turned to Cathy in the first instance for support. The surprise of hearing that Sally was leaving to live with another person was perhaps as big for Cathy as it was for Angus.

Because they knew each other well, the need to be empathic, rather than sympathetic, was paramount for Cathy. It was not up to her to take sides, least of all Angus' side. This would only have meant that she would reinforce an entrenched attitude. What Cathy did have to do was to listen.

She realized that people who have been shocked and traumatized need to talk about the events surrounding the event causing the shock. Cathy and Angus talked about the help needed by him and the help given by her, and they decided that they would meet every week for four weeks. After that they would review the situation. Cathy also realized that these meetings would not be meetings for counselling, but for listening: in the state in which Angus was then, counselling was not possible. But she could let him talk, and this would lay the groundwork for further work later on. After the first four weeks they went on to meet for six more times at fortnightly intervals.

During the early weeks Angus insisted that he still loved his wife and would have her back any time. But he also readily called her names which he found himself surprised even to know. He could not understand that he was able to say both things sometimes in the same sentence. Cathy listened to him without criticizing him, saying that such confusion is quite normal. Once Angus could see that this is confusion, not madness, he was more at ease, at least for a day or so. Then stronger feelings still presented themselves. When he saw Sally's clothes, he hated her. He had worked so that she could buy some of her clothes; now he resented the money he had given her. The boy looked very much like her, and when he looked at him he reminded him of Sally, and he felt a deep longing for her. His love turned to anger and back again.

These are not the ways in which Angus described what was

going on, but more the words of Cathy, as she told the story, and as she reflected to him what she experienced as happening in his world. As she said some of these things to him, he could relate them to his situation, and many times he said 'ah, yes, that's it'. In his state he may often not have been able to give names to feelings, but gradually, because Cathy recognized the feelings as he described them, Angus became able to notice also what was happening. After a number of meetings, Angus began to feel more in charge and began to recognize that what he was doing at the moment was 'enduring to live' (see Chapter 7). This, they both recognized, was an important meaning in his life because it really meant 'enduring to live so that the children have a home'. While this was both a meaning and a goal for him at this moment, he also decided that a future goal would be not just to survive, but to 'live' again, and this meant a new relationship. As Cathy worked with Angus, she mentioned some of the stages described by Kübler-Ross (see Chapter 2), and this helped him to see his predicament in perspective. The empathic way of being and helping which Cathy represented meant that Angus could cope, and in fact coped and adjsuted remarkably well to his new life. He acknowledged Cathy's help all the time in later meetings, and even after they had finished, his Christmas card to Cathy was always the first to arrive, which Cathy took as a sign of gratitude.

Being empathic with Sheila

The nurse who had mentioned to Sheila that she was separating from her husband might have said this simply in the way that two people in similar situations compare notes. She might not have realized that, by saying this, she was actually giving Sheila an opportunity to explore her past and her left-over feelings. In fact, the nurse showed empathy in that she noticed that Sheila mentioned 'guilt' a few times. This had in fact surprised Sheila; she had never given this much concentrated thought. She experienced guilt, but never called what she experienced by that name. The fact that the nurse heard the word and said it helped Sheila to trust the nurse: she seemed a genuine (congruous) person. The fact that the nurse was also honest by saying that she was willing but that she was not a trained counsellor made her even more genuine.

By picking up the fact that Sheila felt guilt, and saying so, the nurse put herself into that 'private perceptual world of the other', 'moving about in it delicately without making judgements'. The nurse said that she noticed the word 'guilt' a few times. By saying so she simply made a statement; she did not make this as a judgement, nor did she challenge Sheila to either agree or disagree. It is this way of being with another person which makes a person either empathic or not. The choice of the words, the way she looked at Sheila, the tone of her voice, the stance of her body – all these elements go together to convey that one cares.

There may be many ways of saying what empathy is, and perhaps all of us have different ways of saying it at different times and in different circumstances. What matters is that we recognize when we are empathic or not; for the other person perceives much more quickly than we if there is empathy present or not. When we can learn to know our own level of being with others, then we can also change if we want to.

People who are bereaved because of some loss in their lives may be confused and hurt, but they are also very acutely aware of the behaviour of others towards them. People who have been bereaved – be this through death or divorce – have been wounded, and when a wound is raw and open it is painful when it is being touched wrongly. This indicates that those who want to help the bereaved and those grieving separation and loss, need to know something of the feelings and circumstances of such events. It does not mean that only people who have been bereaved can help the bereaved, and only those who have been divorced can help the divorced, but it does mean that those who want to help have to have some sense of what is going on in the private perceptual world of those they are trying to help. Reading about such events helps, but we can also achieve much with imagination. But perhaps simply being ourselves – being empathic – helps most. However short an encounter or a helping situation, the relationship which will have existed for that time will have been the vehicle for change and adaptation.

Further reading

Doyle, R. (1996) *The Woman Who Walked Into Doors*. London: Jonathan Cape.

Feeney, J. and Noller, P. (1996) *Adult Attachment*. London: Sage.

Weldon, F. (1996) *Splitting*. London: Flamingo.

CHAPTER NINE

Loss of a career and security
Listening

....

Kingsley was 46 and enjoyed his work as the manager of a large hospital in a northern town. He felt capable, and pleased that he had reached this position at a relatively young age. He had worked hard for this job, wanting to give his family both here and in Jamaica a sense of achievement and freedom from the grind which he had known in his youth. He had also successfully steered his hospital through the application for trust status. Now only one major hurdle was still there: the merger with another hospital, much smaller than his, for purposes of administration. He felt confident that all was going well. In his discussions with the health authorities he had picked up the unspoken promise that he would be heading the new team. There seemed no question about it. When the day came for signing the deal, he was called to the chairman's office and emerged after a short while, with a letter of dismissal in his hand. The manager of the other hospital had been appointed the new head.

Not unreasonably, Kingsley was not just shocked at this decision, he also sensed discrimination and unfairness. The other man was white, younger, and a local person.

Kingsley went to his office and closed the door. He found it hard to cry, and indeed he could not cry, such was his shock. His thoughts were a jumble of anger, disappointment, guilt for having been so confident, shame and defeat. His secretary finally summoned up enough courage to join him. She did not have to ask what had happened – it was written all over Kingsley's body and the air was full of it. She poured them both a whisky and sat with him for a long time, neither of them speaking. Gradually, as she sat next to Kingsley, she began to hear some of what was going on inside him. She said little more than 'mmh' and 'yes', but this helped Kingsley to get some grip on his situation, at least enough to feel that he could go home that evening.

Months later, and with much help from staff and friends, Kingsley got compensation for unfair dismissal. Eighteen months later he had another job, but the time in between was one of 'going into hell', as he put it.

Moira was in hospital to have her bunions done. On the second evening postoperatively, Edgar, a staff nurse, found her sitting in the chair beside her bed, quietly weeping. When he went up to her, she said she had a lot of pain. She had had some medication only recently, and before she had not appeared to be in the kind of pain which makes one cry. Edgar guessed that something was not as it should be, and he put his arm around her, asking what was troubling her.

Moira dried her tears and said that it was the anniversary of her husband's death. Edgar expressed his sympathy, thinking that it was perhaps the first anniversary. Then Moira volunteered that it was the 20th anniversary of his death. Edgar registered surprised, but tried not to show this. Instead, he said, 'tell me about your husband'. It was just as well that he had time, because this opening was just what Moira was looking for. She told him a long story.

Moira's husband (she never mentioned his name) had been a career diplomat, and they had spent most of their time in the Far East. When he was 52 and Moira was 50, he had a heart attack and died while they were on a tour. Had they been nearer to medical help, he might have survived. For Moira, his death meant the loss of a role, a house, an income, and most of all, she had to move back to England to get what pension she was entitled to. Having two sons at university meant that she had to consider earning for herself: not easy for someone who until then had relied on domestic help and was used to a rather lavish life-style. Moira found work as an assistant in a flower shop. She loved this, because she was still in touch with people with money.

Being on her feet all day made her bunions grow. She had put on a brave face in order to support herself in this rather lowly way, and she often had memorable parties in her bedsit, squeezing in as many people as she could. She had never entirely adjusted to her 'fall from grace', as she so poignantly called it. Twenty years later the loss of her status and life-style was as painful as it ever was. She blamed her husband for leaving her without warning and preparation. Harbouring a grudge had somehow kept her alive. Now, the pain from the operation touched on the pain in her soul.

The loss of a career

Unemployment and loss of jobs are such daily events in our lives that we have came to live with the idea. Indeed, employment is now often considered more like good fortune than either a right or a fact of life.

Many of the family names in Western countries refer to someone's trade or profession, by which they were presumably identified. In our society, men and women are generally identified by what they *do*, rather than by who they are. While it is no longer a stigma to have to say, when asked, 'I am unemployed', the mere word 'unemployed' hints that 'employed' is the norm. This also means that generally we think of people being employed by others. Self-employment is still often considered risky. We tend to think of tradespeople as self-employed: window cleaners, plumbers and builders. But people with university degrees and diplomas take risks when using their qualifications independently. When people are asked what they do, in conversation or on forms, one is expected to say or write one word. Self-employed people with a 'portfolio of jobs', that is, pursuing several careers or occupations at once, find themselves in another dilemma: which one to mention? Perhaps 'portfolio' working may become the norm for the future, absorbing some of the shocks from loss of jobs.

Raphael (1984, p. 300) points out that never will have a job been better and more positive than when it is lost. All the negative aspects of a job may be forgotten when it is no longer there. However much we may have grumbled and hated work, when it is gone it is most desirable and wanted.

When and where large industries or works have closed or 'down-sized' and large numbers of people have lost jobs, the shock may be dampened somewhat. At least there is some safety in numbers, and many other people are in the same position. People who will normally have associated outside of work, meeting in pubs, or playing games or making music together, may still be able to do this. When only some people are laid off, there is a division between the 'in' and the 'out' group which can arise, but when there are many together of either group, the divisions may be less hard to bear.

It is a fact that in recent years it has been men who are made redundant while women have found employment. The traditional roles of men as providers and women as carers of family and home are thus turned upside down. Many women have work, even if it is not well paid, but men find it difficult to take on caring roles and perhaps now live on the salaries which their wives and partners bring home. This scenario may mean that women find themselves newly liberated with a new sense of self-worth. This may have changed the relationship

with their men already. If the men now find that they also
have to take on a different role, they may not only not be
happy, but may resent their whole situation. Changing the
roles also means changing attitudes, and this may not be easy.
When a relationship is therefore not very stable, there may
be disillusion, emotional disengagement, and perhaps a hardening of stereotypes, leading to broken homes, broken families and broken personalities.

This is perhaps a worst-case scenario, and many situations
are not on such a downward spiral. Perhaps after some time
there are other possibilities for new and different jobs. This
means that the time of bereavement for a job is not prolonged,
and the adaptation to a new and different life is made more
or less easily. When this is not possible, the signs of prolonged
grief may become very visible.

Bartley and Fagin (1990) point out that '(i)nterest in the
effect of unemployment on health has declined'. We have
taken for granted that unemployed people are more likely to
be ill and that society as a whole suffers from the effects of
unemployment. It is not only psychiatric illnesses which
increase when someone is unemployed, but circulatory disorders, stress, accidents and smoking-related illnesses are all
increased, as are headaches, sleeplessness, depression, and
exacerbation of dermatological, gastrointestinal and rheumatic
conditions. Child abuse and separations also increase. Alcohol
and drug dependence increase. These illnesses and disorders
cannot be overlooked or dismissed as irrelevant.

Clark (1985) describes losses associated with change in job
status: loss of self-esteem and of nurturing, and loss caused
by the separation. These losses are damaging to the person
and the personality, and can in due course also lead to physical illness.

Losing a job may not be identical with losing a career. Many
health care workers have lost jobs in recent years and have
been able to move to other jobs. But equally many will also
see such an event as an opportunity to leave the health service
altogether. Anecdotal evidence exists in plenty of nurses who
were made redundant and are now working as secretaries or
in shops. These people did not have the emotional stamina
to fight their way around the system. This is not surprising;
in today's job market the competition is very tough.

The feelings caused by a job loss

When someone does unexpectedly lose a job, the feelings which are engendered are not dissimilar to those of someone unexpectedly bereaved.

Raphael (1984, p. 300) mentions that usually there is shock, numbness and disbelief. These are the well-known responses of bereaved people everywhere. With the loss of the job goes the loss of colleagues and workmates, security and self-esteem. When there is no possibility of finding similar work again, the loss of these elements is perhaps even harder to bear.

When someone finds himself or herself not needed any more, there is the sense of being dispensable, only good for the scrap heap. After years of service to an employer, there is now an experience of rejection which hits to the core. Perhaps someone younger has got the job: one has become useless. Perhaps someone more skilled is wanted: one's experience does not count. Perhaps the experience of being sidelined for someone younger, or for a machine or robot, is the ultimate experience of rejection. Because we identify with our work, when work disappears, we disappear, in a manner of speaking.

The feelings which go with such a situation are not difficult to imagine: helplessness, inadequacy, impotence, purpose-lessness, shame, rage, and uselessness. Realistically, it may be that there are very sound reasons for making someone redundant, but for the person concerned, cool rationality may not be very helpful. For that person it is a matter of being or non-being – at least while the state of shock, numbness and disbelief lasts.

Feelings of envy of other people who have not been similarly dismissed, and hatred of those who dismiss, can be very strong. When such feelings are not acknowledged and worked with, they can easily form the beginning of a destructive course of chronic grief, characterized by bitterness and anger.

The same kind of searching for the cause which goes on when a beloved person dies also goes on when someone is made redundant. What was the reason? Did the person not perform well enough? Should there have been more effort to learn new skills, and more interest in taking a lead or changing? Chapman (1989, p. 24) gives an example of two men, Colin and Mark, who were both in line for promotion, but had to wait a while yet. Mark 'used the waiting period to improve relationships and hone his skills. Colin, on the other hand, became discouraged and let things slip'. Mark was promoted, but Colin was told that he disqualified himself by not staying involved. Should Colin have been told what to do before the event? It seems rather unfair of management to watch a situation and not help. This may be a fictitious scenario, but in real life such situations may lead to resentment and feelings of anger at not being treated equally.

Unlike death, many situations of loss of job have the possibility of redress. Unfair dismissal for various reasons (in the case of Kingsley for racial reasons) can be pursued. This takes much energy and patience, and the outcome may not be assured or be satisfactory. In the early stages, however, the energy from strong feelings of anger and frustration may be directed into fighting to get back what was lost, or to get redress. This generally needs some help, but it can also help a person to cope with what happened. This path is not normally open to people who have been made redundant when factories or works close. Their redundancy payments may however be some form of compensation.

Listening to what is happening

It is the province of knowledge to speak and it is the privilege of wisdom to listen
(O.W. Holmes, 1872, *The Poet at the Breakfast Table*).

Sometimes when writing about a subject, I go through the subject indexes of many books, looking for the relevant topic. More often than not I am disappointed, by not finding the topic in books where I had expected it, but finding it in others where perhaps I might not have expected it. I did this with the word 'listening', looking for it in the books so far quoted in this text. I was astonished by how many books on bereavement do not mention the word in their index.

When we want to help someone – and we are in the 'helping professions' to help – then the first real means of helping we have is to listen. It may even be true to say that in order to be human, to be a person, we have to listen. We can only be a person when we interact with other persons. If we want to be human in the widest sense, then we also interact with the whole of creation. We have a certain relationship with dandelions as well as waterfalls, simply because we share the planet with them. Our way of interacting with this creation is by listening. We are made human when we respond to the world around us. Responding means that we have heard something interpreting it and giving an answer. Or we may see a colourful tree and feel delight. We may unexpectedly see a pair of eyes at night and be afraid. Listening is not simply making the ears work, but being aware of all that goes on around us.

When we want to help another person, we have to hear what that person has to say. Certainly, not many words may need to be spoken. The secretary in Kingsley's story did not speak much, but she heard him deeply and responded to his need.

One of the reasons for putting the model for helping in the form of questions is so that a story can be told. This implies that the person who asked the question can listen and is willing to listen. It means having time to listen, and also giving the attention which is perhaps the first prerequisite to helping. We cannot listen when we are really thinking of a lot of other things.

The first question, 'what is happening?' is the question of the person who wants to listen and to hear. Listening and 'what is happening' are almost synonymous. When we see a need we ask, 'what is happening?'. When we try to find out what is going on, we have to listen to the story which has to be told at that moment.

The quote from Rogers (1980) on empathy in the last chapter continues (p. 143):

To be with another in this way means that for the time being, you lay aside your own views and values in order to enter another's world without prejudice. In some sense it means that you lay aside yourself; this can only be done by persons who are secure enough in themselves that they know they will not get lost in what may turn out to be the strange and bizarre world of the other, and that they can comfortably return to their own world when they wish.

Two pages further on (p. 145) Rogers quotes a manual which has been prepared for ordinary people who want to help particularly those who live in the alienated counter-culture chaos of large cities. The manual is very specific: 'You only listen and say back the other person's thing, step by step, just as that person seems to have it at that moment. You never mix it into any of your own things or ideas'. Rogers concludes by saying that 'it seems clear that an empathic way of being, although highly subtle conceptually, can also be described in terms which are perfectly understandable by contemporary youth or citizens of a beleaguered inner city' (p. 146). This kind of listening is empathic, and being empathic means listening in a radical way to what is happening now, to this person.

The
components of
listening

Listening is the first of the helping and counselling *skills* described here. The other skills specifically mentioned are reflecting (see Chapter 10), goal setting (see Chapter 11) and challenging (see Chapter 12). For helping in any situation and at any stage of the helping process, listening is necessary. It does not mean that listening is specifically needed in situations of loss of job; it simply means that listening is here applied particularly to this type of loss. This section also applies to all the other situations described in this book – and to those encountered in real life by the readers.

Listening is not just for the ears, but involves the whole of the setting of an encounter for helping. Burnard (1994, p. 114) describes three aspects of listening:

Linguistic aspects of speech which refer to the actual words which the person uses, the words, phrases and figures of speech, as well as the forms of expression and metaphors used which are personal.

Paralinguistic aspects which include the timing, volume, tone, pitch, fluency, range and the 'fillers' like 'um' and 'er'.

Non-verbal aspects such as facial expression, gestures, body position, body movements, eye contact, etc.

Burnard warns that helpers should be careful not to interpret or assume too much, but check with the client if this is really what he or she might be feeling or thinking. Perhaps again, rather than saying 'I see that you are uncomfortable', it may be better to say, 'What is happening at the moment?' and let the other person give the answer or explanation, and let the helper listen.

When we listen to someone, we hear the words spoken, but we also hear the whole person. By paying attention to the non-verbal and the paralinguistic aspects we hear the words in context. We take in what is thus presented, and in and through our person we interpret this and then respond. So that this interpretation can be accurate we have to have a good sense of self-awareness and self-knowledge. With these two aspects we are able, paradoxically, to 'lay aside our own views and values' and even lay aside our own selves. This does not mean denying our feelings and experiences at that moment, but it means not referring to them for our own use. Burnard (1994, p. 116) calls this noting our own feelings 'as a guide to the client's feelings'. We are concerned with the response we give, which has to be accurate and helpful. When we can respond accurately we do not only help the other person, but we are helped too, in that we have gained some understanding for ourselves, too. This is what makes helping so satisfying and so demanding. Ideally, in a helping situation such moments happen many times.

We can create the climate in which listening is fostered by several, mostly practical, means. Some of those have been described in more detail in Chapters 6–8. Perhaps the most basic aspect is that we actually want to listen. When we *have* to listen, we may do so reluctantly. All nurses (and all people) have again and again used words like 'of course I want to listen to you' while inwardly groaning that we have to hear the same old story again. This is very human, but perhaps not very congruent. If in saying 'of course I want to listen to you' we actually give ourselves permission to mean what we say, we will also have listened to ourselves. Equally, we may have to say 'I don't have time to listen now, but I will come back shortly' (or give some other stated time). This may not only be honest and congruent, but also empathic and respectful of both people in the relationship.

Effective listening means being relaxed, and being more or less at the same level as the other person. There should be no big objects like desks etc. between the two people. We need to maintain eye contact and convey to the other that only he or she matters at the moment by our posture and perhaps by our words.

Listening also means *listening* and not talking, not interrupting, not interpreting, being comfortable with silence when indicated, and using prompts like 'go on' etc. to encourage the other person to continue talking.

We stop listening when we try to finish sentences for the other, become aware of our needs which need attention, when we are tired or bored, begin to think more about the next task, or when we find that we have such a similar problem that we are no longer empathic but begin to sympathize, or when we become frightened that we cannot handle a situation or have no experience. In such situations often the best thing to do is to focus attention on the self for just a moment, take stock, and perhaps admit to the problem. When we can do that, then the other person will usually understand. If we try to go on regardless, the client will soon enough find that the attention has gone and may become irritated and feel let down. Listening is not easy. It is 'a way of being' with another person which is demanding. But when we listen we give of our best and we receive the best.

Listening to the bereaved

Listening to the bereaved is not more difficult than listening to people in other situations. Perhaps the main difference is that the bereaved often have an immense need to talk. They also often need to tell their story many times over. Even if we have heard it before, and say so, we should be prepared to hear it again.

It is in talking that many people begin to understand what is happening to them. In telling the story it becomes real. Those who have lost someone or something prematurely, unexpectedly and unjustly, need to talk to recognize and access the feelings which have been aroused by the event and the shock thus created. Because the feelings are often so strong, they are also in competition with each other. Feelings of anger and self-pity may follow each other within seconds, the first making one feel ready for a fight, only to be replaced just as quickly by a total sense of helplessness,with all energy drained. The fact that people often experience such opposites in rapid succession can lead them to fear that they are going mad or have lost a sense of reality. Talking and being listened to with unconditional positive regard can help a person to accept that she or he is all right. Just admitting such thoughts and feelings can be helpful. Listening empathically means acknowledging that we have heard, that we are not shocked, and perhaps assuring the person that if he or she were not feeling like this we might be more worried.

Listening to a person who has lost a job often means that we hear indeed all kinds of unsavoury things because the situation is unsavoury. We do not make things right just by listening, but by hearing what the person has to say we give that person an opportunity to deal with feelings as is appropriate at that moment. In the early days of a severe loss there is a need just to talk. Later on there comes the need to make sense, find some meaning, get some order re-established, and begin to adjust. The listening done is helping this process to take shape.

It is an active listening, which means that we have to respond in a skilled way. We have to reflect, challenge and perhaps summarize in such a way that the person can work towards a goal. It should surely be the case that at the end of a helping interaction the person is in a better space than at the beginning. This does not mean that we placate with a 'there, there', but that we respond in some way which is hopeful, supportive and looks forward. Very often this means telling the person in some way that she or he *is* OK, is doing well, has it within himself or herself to adjust and go on. We do this not to make our job easier, but simply because we believe this. Our experience has taught us to believe it, and we may need to share this belief with the person. Perhaps this may mean that that person comes to trust us; if so, we will have listened well. This comes because we have trusted the person with us in the first instance.

Being heard

Most of us will have some memory of a time or an occasion when we felt really heard. Someone listened to us and made us feel accepted. Most of us will also know that such moments are rare and very precious. This is not because they are intrinsically rare, but because most of the time we do not experience the sort of listening which makes such moments happen. These days we can go to a counsellor or similar therapist and be heard, but we normally have to pay for such a service. Some people think that it is good to pay for such a service because it makes us work harder. When we listen as part of another role or job, we do not charge for listening and the experience of being heard comes free.

What is it like for people who are bereaved in some way to be listened to, to be accepted unconditionally, to meet a congruent, empathic person?

If we say that people are empathic rather than use empathy, then the proof of this must be the experience of the person concerned. Debates about whether counselling and psychotherapy actually help anyone are useful, but how can such hypotheses be measured?

The story of Kingsley showed that his secretary's action – going into his room and sitting with him – was crucial to him. Without her action he would not have been able to collect his thoughts enough to go home. There is no way of knowing what else might have happened, but it is possible to guess that Kingsley might have walked out of the hospital leaving behind him a number of confused and hurt people. He might have driven home in a dangerous way, possibly causing an accident. He might have spent an awful evening with his family. The family will still have had to help him, and they will still have had to talk a great deal, but the fact that he was probably over the worst of the shock, will have made these talks more productive. His secretary listened to his behaviour, his non-verbal communication, and maybe also his words, but they were not recorded. That afternoon she was a person of empathy, showing him unconditional positive regard, able to feel at home in his world and laying her own world aside. She was attentive, hopeful and supportive (even pouring a drink). She listened in the only way possible: by being there.

Edgar, the nurse who noticed Moira crying, listened in a different way. He too noticed a non-verbal cue first and responded to that. But then he had to listen to a long story. The fact that the main event happened 20 years ago leaves one to guess that many other people have also had to listen to Moira's story before. But her character suggests that she had managed to suppress her real feelings for most of that time – hence they surfaced now when some other pain woke up the old pain of the grief. This grief may need more attention than Edgar would be able to give Moira in a short time. But the fact that he listened to her in a helpful, therapeutic way, means that he will perhaps have helped Moira to realize that she is not yet through with her grief and might need to look for some help. Once the old grief is woken up it is less easily put down again, and is perhaps now crying out for more attention. The fact that Edgar helped Moira to acknowledge her grief and pain of bereavement may have helped her eventually to lead a more contented life, more realistically within her means, and also, one hopes, more happily.

When we listen to others we give them the gift of humanity; being heard means receiving the gift of personhood.

Further reading   Long, A. (1990) *Listening*. London: Daybreak.

CHAPTER TEN

Loss of a home and property
Reflecting
....

The caravan

The news came, as it so often does, by way of a phone call. The
site owner was embarrassed, then blurted it out. My caravan was
gone; stolen.

My first reaction was almost casual, stoic, thinking only of
insurance claims and informing the police. I filled in forms, sat in
a police station, thinking that it was inconvenient – but also that it
was unusual, new, very real, almost exciting. I was treated as a
victim without experiencing pain. I felt almost guilty – did they suspect me of organizing the theft for insurance purposes?

At the end of the day I set out to go home – but my intention had
been to go to the caravan. There was food waiting in the fridge, my
slippers, casual clothes for the evening, a novel half-read. I suddenly
started to remember other things that I would never see again – a
set of crockery that I had treasured for 20 years, photographs, books,
clothes, particular old items of kitchenware. They had been part of
my life for so long I really couldn't believe that I would not reach
into a drawer somewhere and find them. Driving home, I felt homeless – part of me was somewhere else, and could not be recovered.

There was very little of value in the van – but a large chunk of
myself was gone. It leaves an ache of bereavement. I wonder where
the van is now. Who is living in it? What have they done with my
stuff? Has it been destroyed? Is someone else using those cups and
plates in which I invested so many memories?

I told myself to let go, accepting that nothing is forever; but I still
long to find those items again. Even now, months later, when I need
something and go to fetch it, I suddenly remember that it has gone,

and feel – not quite pain, nor anger, but a kind of sudden emptiness. I have bought a new van; new cups; new clothes. But they will never replace what is lost. I am in danger of determining never again to become attached to things – but that would be a shame.

(M.T.)

Alister's parents had bought him a big flat as a wedding present. It was in a suburb, had a wonderful view, easy access to public transport and shops and there were good neighbours. But the marriage did not last, and five years later he began to have lodgers to use some of the space and to help supplement his income. He himself pursued his career as a painter. After his parents had died he began thinking about going to live with friends who formed the nucleus of a therapeutic community. This would mean renting a small, purpose-built house in the complex. He sold his flat easily enough and moved into the new house. But once there, he began to have misgivings. He was not suited to community living and working. The other members found him as difficult as he found them irritating. But he had committed himself. He began to regret his move intensely. He began to feel guilty for selling the flat which his parents had given him. He had made two bad moves, one out and one in. To move back into his neighbourhood was almost impossible. He had no appetite for painting, and therefore had little income. After a year of increasing unhappiness, everyone decided that it would be best if Alister left again. Now he had no home, no career, no self-confidence, and not enough money to buy another decent flat. He hired a car to go house-hunting. One day, looking at a sign rather than the road, he collided with another car. Neither driver was seriously hurt, but the cars were badly damaged. This was yet another loss. His GP gave him the opportunity to talk, and they met on a number of occasions, for which Alister was always grateful.

Losing a home

The prophet, in Gibran's book of the same name (1926, p. 38) says

Your house is your larger body.

And according to Coke (1628)

a man's house is his castle (and each man's home is his safest refuge).

I am writing this chapter a few days after the cold and freeze of Christmas 1995. In the rapid thaw which followed, many people were not only left with broken pipes, but with badly damaged houses due to flooding. Stories of cold houses with sodden furniture and clothes and damaged goods and machinery are in the news for various different reasons.

Everyone who has lost a house or part of a house due to fire, water, storm, earthquake, or other accidental damage, is aware how much one's house and home means. As so often, when we lose it, we become conscious of how important something is. Most of us invest a great deal of money, time and effort into making a house, flat, or room into a 'home'. The 'larger body' spoken of by Gibran gives that impression of extension of ourselves. A home is also that part of ourselves which we can usually easily share with others. We invite people to come to our home to share something of ourselves with them. When the home is lost or destroyed, we have also lost that capacity to share.

Whether we want to or not, we have all been subjected to news of wars and destruction in the world around us. Pictures of families fleeing their homes with little more than what they could carry have invaded our homes. Some of the people who were affected by the earthquake in Kobe, Japan, in 1994 will be traumatized for years after the event. To see pictures of such events may make us very uncomfortable in our comfortable homes. The sense that we can do little about atrocities and destruction inevitably makes us more aware of other people's suffering. A sense of guilt will have come over all of us at some stage: guilt at our helplessness and smugness. It may also have helped us to be more compassionate and understanding.

Most people grow up in a home which then represents some stability for them. People who do not have a home also lack other important things for personal growth and development, such as family and friends or support. Those who do not have the ability to care for a home often find that they do not care for themselves either.

There are many people in all societies who have chosen not to have a home, or not to have a permanent home. Many people the world over are also made homeless by systems and governments of various kinds, and for many reasons such people become burdens for societies. 'Living rough' was once a choice for a minority of people, but it has now become a symbol of lost youth and the degeneration of caring as a valued quality of social buoyancy.

The place where most of the time was spent when we grew up will always hold special memories. It is the place *par excel-*

lence which we normally refer to as 'home'. This place will also be associated with special memories. It has been said that when we lose a parent we lose part of our history; the same could be said when we lose our home: we lose part of our history with the home. Most people accept this as part of life and adjust to it, but however well we are adjusted, it remains an important factor in our lives. We are shaped as much by our home(s) as by many other people, objects and events in our lives.

The homes which Alister 'lost' had specific meanings for him: the first home was given him by his parents and he felt an obligation to them. But it was also the home in which his marriage did not succeed, and this brought feelings of inadequacy to the fore. Then going to the community and selling the house reinforced these two aspects of guilt and self-doubt. Finally, he also lost a lot of money in the various transactions, and he felt he had squandered the gifts given him by his parents. In middle age he was faced with a need to reappraise his entire life. The move out of his house therefore precipitated also the move out of a life-style, values, and attitudes. He grieved for all these things, and only when he was helped to see them as part of a whole process could he begin to settle down again.

Losing a community

When people move house and move to a new place, they will generally know very few people there. They will not necessarily lose the friends they had, but the circle of acquaintances will change. Many people find that moving into certain locations is like moving into foreign territory. Some people find that even after years living somewhere, they are still considered the 'newcomers' or 'outsiders'. Moving home may therefore not just be the exciting, joyful and challenging move which was anticipated. Moving home may be a move into hostility. It is therefore not surprising that some people become disillusioned and apathetic. In such a state they may withdraw into their 'castle', pull up the drawbridge, and stay isolated. The move may have been not just a move, but a loss.

There are many ways of losing a community which had been supportive. Alister had joined a community of a special kind, hoping that this would support him as a single person. But such a community existing for a specific purpose might also be exclusive for those who do not share their ideals. Joining a community may mean an enormous investment for a person, and then to be excluded again may truly be considered a loss of identity.

The religious communities to which people belong are often of unmeasurable significance. Ties of friendship and sharing of faith may have been built up for many years. In particularly, elderly people who move into homes away from their residence may find that they lose a vital part of their lives. They may not make friends easily and losing the spiritual ties with a whole set of people can be a source of deep grief.

Some religious communities exclude members who do not conform to strict rules. For instance, some Jehovah's Witnesses will exclude their members if they have willingly or unwillingly received blood products. At a time of stress and illness such an action may be particularly hard to bear and turn people against any religion altogether.

Children who change school often find that they miss their friends. This may not last too long, but it should never be underestimated. The trauma which may be caused by repeated changes of school may not always be evident just at the time, but may cause serious problems with relationships in later life. The unfinished grief of such situations can accumulate and later on manifest as emotional pain and perhaps also as mental illness.

Losing property

There can be hardly anyone who has not lost property at some stage. Whether this happens through theft, accident, or carelessness, there is generally a sense of hurt, anger, and perhaps also of guilt. 'If only ...' is the accusation we make to ourselves. We should have been more careful, more thoughtful, less trusting.

Property can usually be replaced, but it is not so easy. The story of the stolen caravan shows well enough that it is not just the things themselves which count, but the value which we give to them.

In earlier years and centuries books, handwritten over many years, could be burned and a life's work lost in an instant. Today, the same is still possible when computers are stolen, or even worse, when computers are left in cars and the cars are stolen.

When the loss of property is caused by theft and burglary, there is often a sense of having been invaded. The 'larger body' has been violated, but the actual body feels it. A burglary is usually a messy affair, with drawers opened and tipped

up and furniture damaged and spoiled. Burglars normally do
their work in very little time, and they do not care how the
people feel after they have gone. The feeling of having been
assaulted, robbed of tangible links with special people, not
just their gifts, and not respected as a person, can leave deep
wounds. Some people feel that they can never trust others
again. They become suspicious and furtive and surround
themselves with many kinds of behaviours and attitudes to
protect themselves emotionally and practically.

The prevalence of disregard of property has also left a
wound in the psyche of nations and people. Not daring to go
out at night, putting everything under lock and key, securing
houses with grilles and fences, have had an impact which may
not always be acknowledged. But we are all part of such trends
and marked by them. There may be a sense of 'it happens to
everyone' and therefore it is easier to tolerate. This is true,
but any intrusion into personal space is suffered differently
by everyone, because it is personal.

Services like 'Victim Support' have been very welcome and
very helpful generally, but not everybody who has been a victim can get this service. However small a loss may be, it is
always significant for the person concerned.

The purpose of helping

When we meet people who are actively or unexpectedly
mourning some loss, we cannot assume that they want to
adjust and let go and live life without the grief. The shock
experienced at first was a defence mechanism for not being
too hurt. When people allow the state of shock to go on, they
may never really face the grief. Perhaps they are afraid of what
they find there.

When a patient, client, colleague or friend specifically asks
for help with a problem, we have a professional duty to help
to the best of our ability. This may often mean that help is
asked for something which may be uppermost but not the
most important problem. The main aspect may emerge only
gradually; it may very often be an unmourned loss or an unac-
knowledged grief.

When we, as helpers, think that someone has a problem
with a loss – perhaps someone in hospital for an operation or
illness and we suspect that there is some deeper worry there –
we have no right to go to that person and say, 'You should
look at your past and come to terms with your loss'. Unless
we have heard a story, we cannot impose our perceptions or
assumptions. But when, in the course of a conversation, we

have perhaps come across some buried grief and it has been noticed, we should try to help the person to become aware of it.

But why? Perhaps the person has coped well enough until now. The story of Moira (see Chapter 9) showed that she had managed for 20 years to live reasonably adequately with her sorrow. Why should we try to interfere?

In recent times there have been debates as to whether counselling and psychotherapy actually help, or if they are a new form of paternalism. Do people who like to influence others become counsellors? These may be salutary considerations which we should keep in mind. There are two possibilities for guarding against imposing our views on others or making others deal with memories, feelings and emotions which should either not be dealt with, not yet, or not in this way: using a model such as that proposed in this book, based on questions; and concentrating on the person, not the problem.

There are other safeguards, too, against the possibility of going on an ego-trip as helpers:

being aware of our limitations
being aware when we may be less empathic
being aware when we are no longer unconditionally positive in our regard of clients
when we talk rather than listen
when we as helpers follow our agenda rather than the client's agenda.

Perhaps the next most effective way of safeguarding the client's right, space and integrity is asking

Would you like me to help you?
How can I help you?

'Helping' is there for the other person, not for ourselves. When we use the skills adequately, we are much less prone to fall into the traps of giving advice and telling others who or what they should be. The skill of reflecting is one of the best and most effective skills of helping, and this will be considered next.

Reflecting the meaning of it

The basis of empathy is that we hear and understand what the other person is saying and feeling, and that we let the other know that we have understood this. It is not enough that we have noticed some pain, feeling or need; we have to put it to the person concerned in such a way that she or he is aware that we have heard it. The skill of reflecting helps us to do this. The question 'what is the meaning of it?' is both a question to be asked of the other person and a question which, as helpers, leads us to be empathic.

You say that you are well, but I hear a hesitation in your voice.
You have accepted that you are limited, and I believe you. I simply sense that there is something else there which bothers you.
You said that with a feeling which I had not heard before.

The skill of reflecting consists of two layers:

1) the person's actual words are repeated, but perhaps in a different tone of voice:

Client: I have always looked after my home very well.
Helper: *You* always looked after your home?

This simple repetition of the words helps to keep on the subject presented by the client. As a skill, it is very useful in establishing contact and in helping the client to tell the story. It moves the process of helping on, but in small steps, which may be the pace needed at that moment.

2) Something from the client's non-verbal or paralingual repertoire is reflected:

Client: I am so ashamed having to admit this.
Helper: It seems as if there are lots of other feelings there as well.

Here the helper may have noticed something in the client's eyes, voice, posture, or the context in which a particular phrase is spoken. The empathy (see Chapter 8) which gives a helper the possibility to move in the other's world, now gives the helper the possibility to point out what also seems to be there in this world. It is a reflective response which guides to the meaning. It may be that the helper has sensed something of the wider meaning which the other is either implying or not quite seeing, and rather than give the entire meaning, the helper puts it in such a way that the other person can make the connection.

When such responses are offered perhaps tentatively or as questions, the client can accept them. They are not judgements or accusations. When they are phrased as coming from the helper (*I* hear a hesitation; *I* sense that there is something else; *I* had not heard you say that before) there is also more of a possibility that the client can say no to the suggestion. Were it said as:

You were not sure there
There is more there than you admit
You never said that before

the client may have to defend himself or herself and may more easily feel pressured or accused. By themselves these last statement may be very legitimate reflections, but they may not be helpful ones. Reflection therefore is not just a skill of repeating what was said or what was noticed; it is also a skill of basic communication.

The skill of reflecting is very wide-ranging. We can reflect aspects of exploration, we can seek new information, reflect feelings, body language, perceptions, meanings, goals and ideas. Some people express themselves in terms of words, others in term of images. It is often good to pay attention to such significant expressions and perhaps highlight a word, which then can lead further:

Client: I just seem to be going along like a snail these days.
Helper: A snail?
Client: Yes, you know, carrying my house and everything on top of me.
Helper: That is an interesting image. Say a bit more about this snail.
Client: Well, a snail also leaves a silvery trail.
Helper: What does that mean for you?
Client: I make an impact where I go.

With reflection we can help people to understand themselves and their situation better, perhaps seeing a meaning even in small and insignificant events and expressions. We do not push the understanding, but we push the person's own capacity to tap the understanding which is essentially there already.

The skill of reflection is always a step towards 'what is the meaning of it?'. The question itself may still have to be asked directly, but when looking for the sense, purpose or meaning in a thought, an action, a memory or an event or state, being reflectively skillful will be most helpful.

How do we best help a bereaved person?

When we have established that there may be a problem with coming to terms with a past or present – or even anticipated – loss, we will need to make some mental note of where the client is in the grieving process. It is a good bet that the client is somewhere in the middle of any process, that is, experiencing a growing awareness (Speck, 1978) or moving between bargaining, depression and denial (Kübler-Ross, 1969). Since the stages are not clear-cut, there may be a good deal of movement between various aspects.

In terms of the Four Questions, the person may be trying to find a meaning for what is happening, but had perhaps never thought of actually asking that question. There may therefore have to be some exploration of the scene first. For this purpose in particular, the skill of reflection is very useful.

When we have the permission and the mandate to help a client, then helping can only mean moving somewhere better, more productive, less painful than the present situation. We need to help the person to move forward, and this is often best expressed in terms of a goal. As we cannot change overnight, we need to move forward in the best way possible, and that may be by small but firm steps, trying out the various aspects encountered. The help we can give is directed toward adjusting to the loss and living beyond the pain of grief.

Perhaps one of the most important ways in which we can help is actually to help the person to acknowledge what is going on. When someone has been bereaved for a long time and seems to need help with it, it may be because that person has simply accepted a state of depression and pain as normal. Pointing out that this may actually hinder life can sometimes come as quite a revelation.

Some people are quite capable of dealing with their own feelings when they have been given the 'handle' that what is going on is a bereavement. Admitting it is the important step.

All the authors (e.g. Penson, 1990; Raphael, 1984; Worden, 1991) who write about bereavement make it clear that the person needs to do three basic things:

Become aware of the grief
Acknowledge it as grief
Let it go.

One cannot let anything go without knowing what one lets go. Therefore the first step is being aware of it. Acknowledging the grief may mean perhaps saying it out loud. This is so often why people need someone to help them: the helper has knowledge of the process and can perhaps make explicit what the client experiences implicitly; the helper may have a word for something which the client cannot name and therefore cannot quite understand; the helper can see connections where the client may only see isolated events. The experience of the helper can help legitimize the experience of the client.

Once some aspect, which may have been causing pain in some dark corner of the psyche, is brought into the light of day, it tends to lose its power. It tends also to lose its need to be there. But it needs to be acknowledged and perhaps talked about and considered from various different points of view. The skills of reflecting may have helped to bring it to the surface, and now the same skill can help it to be seen for what it really is: what is this grief? Sometimes another word or another image can put it into perspective.

When this happens, the next step is to let it go. This has often been described as 'saying goodbye'. People may have buried their loved ones, divorced or separated from some person with whom they had nothing more in common, but the final 'goodbye' may never have been said. This may occasionally be an actual word, or it may be an act. It does not matter how or what it is, as long as the inner experience of letting go is also there. The skill of reflecting may therefore be helpful to guide the person to come to the acknowledgement that an adjustment is necessary.

Reflecting on the loss of a home

The man who has written the account of the theft of his caravan probably did not need any counselling help. But the fact that he wrote his story down means that he was deeply affected by the loss. He realizes that he should let go of possessions, but in order to stay human, he needs to be attached. Letting go is easier said than done. Maybe we need to let go of some things and not of others – and we need to know which to let go of and which to keep.

Alister had lost much more than 'just' a home. His home was not stolen, but in a way he destroyed it himself. The guilt which so often goes with a loss is here reinforced. When someone close to us dies, we usually have some feelings of guilt that we should have done more, or cared better, tried to mend a relationship – or secured the van better. When we have to take all the responsibility for a mistake, though, then the feelings of having let ourselves down can be quite overpowering.

A helper's task is not to apportion blame, nor to judge others. By acknowledging what the person says, we lay the basis from which to work. The client's perceived world in this case was that he had let everybody down, his parents, his neighbours, his friends at the community, and also himself.

The GP who helped him, however, said neither that he was to blame, nor that he was not to blame. She accepted Alister as he was. This acceptance was partly responsible for helping Alister to work through his feelings.

Alister's loss was not a usual bereavement, but there was no doubt that it was nevertheless just that. A home is normally at least in part the place where we form our character and personality. We become ourselves within the structure of bricks and mortar. We become attached to the house and its atmosphere. The memories which a house holds are important. Most people would like to die in their own home. Yet in the Holmes and Rahe (1967) social readjustment scale, 'change in residence' is only given 20 out of 100. This must be because it is considered a fruitful and helpful move. When it is not, it must surely go up in the scale.

Nurses and other health care workers will often meet people who will have struggled to stay in a home, however uncomfortable. Then came the day when they either had an accident or became too ill to stay on. They had to go to hospital and from there they might go to some other place of care. They will have had to adjust to illness or some other loss of function as well as perhaps never seeing their home again. Many people accept this as part of getting old, or being ill, but as nurses and helpers we should not underestimate such losses. Helping others to adjust to the loss must surely be one of the more demanding and sensitive jobs. Many of us are also much younger than our clients, making such a task that much more challenging.

Further reading   Weldon, F. (1983) *The Life and Loves of a She Devil*. London: Hodder & Stoughton.

CHAPTER ELEVEN

Loss of a pet
Goal setting

....

Jo was about 30 and was a very popular administrator in a hospital. He just loved guinea pigs. He had a wonderful male which he called Sunrise, because he was always there to greet him in the morning. This morning he was not there, and Jo quickly noticed him curled up dead in his cage. He took him in his arms and stroked him and secretly hoped that the tears he was weeping over him might revive him. But he was really dead.

Once inside the hospital, Jo told everybody he met. He was so upset that he could not do much intelligent work that morning. The news spread through the hospital that Jo's pet had died, and the reactions were generally either a condescending kind of smile or a matter of fact 'oh'. At least, that was what Jo saw and experienced. The staff in his office bought him a little card with some daffodils on it and wrote 'With Sympathy' on the front and signed it. The card was on Jo's desk for about six months – the time it took him to feel able to buy another male guinea pig.

Commenting on the card one day to him, a nurse asked how he was getting on without Sunrise. Jo looked at her and thought for a moment, then replied 'Thank you for asking. I now know who my real friends are in this hospital'. He meant the ones who did not laugh.

Benjy the rabbit

Benjy was Anna's ninth birthday present and came to us when he was only six weeks old.

From the outset, Anna was extremely fond of him, cleaning out his cage daily, putting him in his run whenever the weather permitted, collecting tit-bits for him and so forth. He was always a character, coming to lie next to us if we were working in the garden and even chasing the children, as a dog would.

When he was nearly two years old, he became ill with an ear infection which affected his balance, so we took him to the vet. Although he went to the vet within hours, his condition had deteriorated quite rapidly and the vet told us he would need daily injections of antibiotics and vitamins for several days.

We brought Benjy's hutch into the house and wrapped him in a hand towel we'd heated on the radiator so he would keep warm, but he was so ill, he just lay on his side. Anna dripped water into his mouth, but he was not interested in anything. Although we did not expect him to survive the night, Anna never gave up hope, merely asking 'when' we thought he would be better.

After his third visit to the vet for his injections, during which time there had been no improvement, we carried him home in his box. As Anna lifted him into his hutch she commented that 'He must be getting better, Mummy, he's done a wee and a poo'. Jerry and I checked him very carefully for several minutes for signs of life but he had obviously just passed away.

Anna stood watching us, just quietly repeating 'He's all right, isn't he?' 'He's getting better, isn't he?' Jerry held her hand and said 'I'm sorry, sweetheart, he's died'.

Anna became hysterical within seconds, shouting 'No, don't say that. Stop lying to me. He's not dead, he's not', but she knew he was, as she would not go and check him for herself. She rushed upstairs and locked herself into the bathroom, sobbing and shouting and flinging herself about. Jerry had to force the bathroom lock and hold her very tightly for a long time before she calmed down at all.

She appeared outwardly to recover quite quickly and by the following day she was merely subdued. Benjy was buried in the garden and she bought two fuchsia plants for his grave as he'd loved eating the leaves. We put his hutch back in the shed and she would talk about him quite happily. She put several pictures of him up in her room.

We didn't realize how deeply she felt Benjy's death for a little while. The first sign was when I was cleaning out her clothing drawers some days later and I found the towel that Benjy had been wrapped in, tucked away at the back. I insisted that it be washed if she wanted to keep it, but she refused to part with it, keeping it in a plastic bag in her room. I eventually washed it and replaced it in the bag without her knowing. It's still there.

Some friends were going on holiday and I offered to look after their rabbit as we had a hutch and a run. Anna overheard the conversation and I found her crying quietly in her room – she couldn't bear the thought of another rabbit in Benjy's hutch and I had to withdraw my offer to our friends. She has quietly and firmly rejected any offers of a new rabbit, even when admiring baby rabbits in pet shops.

Recently, some 15 months after Benjy's death, we needed space in *the shed for new bicycles. Jerry moved Benjy's hutch out onto the concrete area next to the shed. Anna discovered this and it again resulted in silent crying in her room. She can't bear the thought of his things being disturbed. She has very reluctantly settled for the hutch being stored in the cellar, although she has no intention of getting rid of it or getting another rabbit or any other pet.*

(A.S.)

Children losing pets

A child's first sense of real loss may be when a cherished toy is broken. Perhaps even more unsettling is when parents finally take away a child's 'comforter'. This may have been inseparable from the child. It may be a dummy which is finally falling apart after months of being sucked or chewed; or it may be a smelly and dirty blanket which accompanied the child everywhere as a toddler. They become a part of the person, or the pet, like the towel in which Benjy was wrapped, in the story above.

Children often experience death first of all with a pet. They may have seen dead animals before, such as mice and birds, but it is different when their own animal dies. The story of Anna shows clearly that the death of her rabbit affected her more strongly than her parents were aware of and perhaps even admitted.

Children have a great capacity to forget and find new interests. But this should not be overestimated. It depends clearly on the age of the child how the death of a pet is accepted. The counselling help which can be given to children depends on the child and the circumstances. Perhaps it is not so much counselling which a child needs, but sensitive explanation and honest answers to the questions which will inevitably be there. But we should never underestimate the capacity of children to be deeply hurt. All of us have memories of such hurts from childhood, which were perhaps dismissed or ridiculed by adults. Children cannot explain their feelings in the same way as adults do, but they still have feelings.

Learning one's limits as a child is a very important aspect of growing and becoming. Perhaps learning what death is about, and what it means and does or does not give may have to be taught many times over. A child who may be more of an introverted character may have particular needs when it comes to understanding the consequences of a loss. It may also be an opportunity for parents and friends to help a child to see that death is not always simply a disaster, but that it can also lead to new understanding and new ways of experiencing the world.

Pet loss and the elderly

The roles which pets play in the lives of elderly people may be very important. Their pets often 'serve as a major source of affection, intimacy, companionship and nurturance' (Carmack, 1991). The grief which they thus feel when a pet dies can be intense.

When elderly people move into sheltered housing, nursing homes or geriatric wards they are often not allowed to take pets with them. This can be devastating. The story is told of a man whose dog was taken away by force because his council house had a no-pet policy, and the man hanged himself. He could not face life without his companion.

People come to rely on their pets for a variety of reasons. Particularly elderly people, who may become more isolated as the years go by, find that having a pet living with them can relieve the isolation. They provide a purpose in their lives as long as they have to look after an animal. Carmack (1991) describes in some detail how elderly people benefit from pet animals, giving them love, tactile stimulation, a sense of security and companionship. Having to clean, feed or walk an animal gives a structure to the day. They have to take care of themselves in order to take care of the pet. If elderly people have to be hospitalized, they may be more willing to go home if they know that there is an animal waiting at home to greet them and need them. On the other hand, having a pet may make people unwilling to go into hospital in the first place.

When a pet dies, an emptiness can result in a person's life which cannot be filled by anyone else. The sense of being needed is gone:

the social system is disrupted, the structure and regular patterns of interaction are missing. There is not the care to give; there is not the source of affection and companionship. There is not the warmth in the home; there is no one to talk to, to sleep with, to feel important to. The grief is experienced not only in feelings of sadness and mourning, but also in the void and emptiness left by the death of a beloved companion animal (Carmack, 1991).

Many pets have been companions for years, and have perhaps aged with the person, both of them needing medical attention at different times. Sometimes an animal has been a deceased spouse's pet, and thus forms a link with the loved person.

There is then an understandable reluctance to get another pet.

The story of Jo showed another aspect of losing a pet. While it seems reasonable that the loss of a pet for a child or an elderly person is a source of grief, the same is not always considered for a younger adult. The same stoic attitude is forced on them as it often is for any loss. But losing an animal who has been a companion is not like losing a hat. Like humans, animals are unique; hats are mass produced. Perhaps, though, people feel less attached to animals the smaller they are. A horse demands more attention than a goldfish, and therefore will be grieved more. We also tend to be more attached to furry animals, like cats, than to slippery ones, like snakes, even though both can be pets.

There are degrees of mourning the loss of a pet every bit as much as mourning the loss of a person. Depending on the emotional attachment formed, pets can be considered more important than people. A young mother, whose father-in-law was dying at the same time as her children's pet cat, confessed that she felt more sorrow for the cat than the father. She was ashamed to feel this, but admitted it nevertheless. Admitting her feelings may have helped her to know where she stood. Having such feelings is not 'wrong'; what matters is how she deals with the feelings once admitted.

Helping people who have lost a pet

Grief after pet loss is not trivial, and can never be dismissed as such. Perhaps the active role of nurses in helping people to adjust to pet loss is, as in most cases of loss, on an individual basis. Carmack (1991) points out that issues of 'self-concept, motivation, potential for injury to self, social system functioning, adaptation, health promotion, crisis intervention and social support' are all concepts in professional nursing practice which relate directly to loss and grief.

The story of Jo highlights the differing reactions of the people around him, and his perception of them. Those who did not trivialize his pain became his friends. As with other kinds of pain, pain is what the patient says it is. People who trivialize the pain caused by the loss of a pet in others, may trivialize also the loss of a person. One wonders if this would be the same if it happened to them.

When we acknowledge that someone is grieving for the loss of a pet, the same attitudes, skills, processes and theories apply. What differs is the way of working with the person concerned. Jo may have needed little more than a day or two to get over most of his shock, and then begin the work of adjusting to his new situation. But Anna was certainly not over her pain yet six months after the event. It is also possible that she may have needed much more help than she was given. The crying silently in her room may have been a cry for attention. She was a child – but many adults may behave in the same way. They retire into a corner with their pain, giving signals of 'leave me alone', but the crying may indicate that in fact they want help and care. Most of us know how comforting an arm around a shoulder can be at such times. It is not too intrusive, but shows compassion and gives the person the opportunity to speak. Perhaps this time no words need to be exchanged, but perhaps next time it is different. Just because it was like this now does not mean that it will be the same some other time. Grieving is not just one thing, but many different things at different times.

Goal setting – what is your goal?

The helping skills outlined here are those of shaping and goal setting, tying in with the question 'what is your goal?' This skill and question are not necessarily specific to helping someone grieving for the loss of a pet, but they are applicable to all helping situations and relationships, and should therefore be read in context with the other topics discussed in other chapters.

All helping is for a purpose: to feel better, to live better, to be out of the morass, and to cope better. Not only when someone asks for help, but also when we offer help, the aim must be that something will be different – better – at the end. But it is also true to say that arriving is often less important than being on the journey. The aim of helping may therefore be to help people be on the journey, rather than be stuck in some siding; be on a path, rather than in a rut; and to walk on their own legs, metaphorically, rather than be carried by events.

Most of us do not talk to ourselves. We tell a story with the purpose of expressing ourselves, contributing to a debate. In so doing we enhance our humanity. We are rarely consciously thinking, when talking, 'now I am enhancing my humanity'. But that is what is happening. There may be plenty of situations in which humanity is not enhanced, such as abuse and verbal warfare. The goal there may be destruction rather than construction; but it is still a goal.

When therefore we tell our story, we do so either to find some meaning by and in what we are saying, or to contribute something important. In helping encounters the first is probably the more usual. A story has to be told so that the meaning behind the story can be discovered. But that is not enough. We have to do something with the meaning and the insight. This is where the skill of helping to find and set a goal is necessary.

When we help someone we help that person to find a goal, not a result; an aim, not a solution. The goal is something 'lively' with which the person is associated, but a result or solution has more of a 'dead certain' feel about it. But the word itself is less important than what it represents to the person concerned. It may also be important that helper and client make sure that they both mean the same thing when discussing something important, otherwise there may be problems later on.

The helper will therefore indicate at some stage that when some significant element has been reached, this needs to be taken further and acted on. A change is almost always necessary, and mostly it means a change of some attitude. A change in behaviour is easier to achieve and may not need the same background to see the necessity. When a change in attitude is recognized, this will normally mean that the person herself or himself has seen that she or he needs to change. Before then, the attitude has normally been that someone else should change, or circumstances should be different. The insight or meaning may have been that the person has 'seen the light' and recognized that the change cannot be effected in others, only in oneself. But such change does not usually happen overnight. Hence the journey to the goal is so important.

The skill of goal setting can be compared to building a pyramid. The basis is broad and perhaps many-sided. That is, the story has many aspects to it and has to cover much ground to get a clear picture. Gradually, as the story is told, the pyramid begins to be built. But so that the edifice remains a pyramid, the helper has to ensure that it is guided towards the top. In practice that means shaping, summarizing, bringing back to the main point, guiding: but always to the client's own goal. This is why the question 'what is your goal?' may have to be asked many times in different ways. A client may not know what he or she actually wants. It may emerge only in the talking, and by reflecting significant words, insights, or phrases and images that a goal may become apparent. This goal needs perhaps to be stated and re-stated several times. Like the builder, when the client may veer off the construction of the pyramid, the helper may need to ask, 'is this still your goal?'

It is possible that the goal may change, or that other, smaller or nearer goals may become apparent. This is very legitimate and helpers who are skilful can help clients to re-formulate goals. But when goals have once been recognized, they should not be abandoned without good reason.

It may be that a person who has lost a pet will say that in three months she wants to buy another pet, and that this is a good goal. It may be a realistic time to wait for the attachment to the dead animal to be loosened and the mind prepared for another pet. But if a week later the person is adamant that she needs another cat now, this may indicate not just a change of mind, but that some other element has appeared which may not have been there before. By helping the client to see what is going on, it is possible to reassess the situation and either change the existing goal or return to it with more understanding.

The skill of goal setting may often be best considered with a series of questions, such as:

Is that what you are looking for?
Are there other problems here?
Are you sure that this is what you want?
What might you regret if you took this road?
What other help might you need?
Is this the best way to follow?

Again, these are not necessarily the actual questions to ask, but if they are not asked as such, a process will need to take place in which the material to be covered by them is included.

Strictly speaking, the skill of goal setting is the client's skill, rather than the helper's. It is the client who needs to identify and set the goal. The helper has to support and encourage the client in keeping to the goal. In terms of goals which bereaved people may have, the most common would probably be to adjust to life without the deceased person, the lost house, job, pet or ideals.

Living with loss

Stating the goal as 'living with loss' will hopefully indicate that the goal is not a 'getting over it'. Many people feel that getting over implies drawing a line under a certain part of life and saying, 'that was it, I must forget about it'. This is neither possible nor desirable. What has happened is part of us and we cannot forget it. Nor can we forget a loved person or object. But we can integrate the memories and use them positively to live in a different mode from now on.

Kushner (1986, pp. 88–9) describes a dinner when someone

said to him, 'How lucky you are to have lost a child when you were so young, so that you could learn to conquer grief and pain. Most people don't have an opportunity like that until they are much older'. Kushner does not give an exact answer, but writes, 'I looked at him incredulously. ... I did not feel lucky to have lost a son whom I loved, neither had I achieved tranquillity or transcended the pain. The sense of loss still hurts years later, though I have learned to live with it'. If we do not experience the pain of loss we will probably not have experienced the joy of living.

Worden (1991, pp. 10–18) describes four tasks of mourning (see Chapter 2) and also four goals of grief counselling (p. 38):

1) *To increase the reality of the loss*
2) *To help the counselee deal with both expressed and latent affect*
3) *To help the counselee overcome various impediments to readjustment after the loss*
4) *To encourage the counselee to say an appropriate goodbye and to feel comfortable reinvesting back into life.*

Rando (1984, p. 18) describes only three tasks, but these are very similar:

1) *Emancipation from the bondage of the deceased*
2) *Readjustment to the environment in which the deceased is missing*
3) *Formation of new relationship.*

When considering the story of Anna above, it seems that she needed to have gone through these same three steps after the death of her pet. In fact, it is possible to substitute 'deceased' for any of the topics discussed in this book, including also the feelings, emotions and 'affects' which go with loss. Perhaps Speck's (1978, p. 12) word 'resolution' covers most of the ideas in these tasks.

The language used by Rando seems stark at first: 'emancipation from the bondage of the deceased'. But when considering this aspect, it is perhaps very apt. When a person continues to grieve, there is a bond created which can easily turn into bondage. This can sometimes be seen in divorce also. Even when a couple had little else in common than perpetual rows during their time together, when one of them leaves, the other may swear that she or he loves him or her absolutely. The marriage bond may have been loose, but the bondage now created around oneself can become so strong that nothing short of drastic action can help. It is natural that what is lost is treasured more now that it is gone than when it was there. The reality of the loss has to be experienced, acknowledged, but then let go.

The steps thus described form a kind of journey: the journey to the goal of establishing a new identity – one without the lost object – creating a new role in life, and altering the self-image to fit the new identity and role. The goal may be to arrive at this new identity. Some people say that one day they wake up and feel different; others may have to tell themselves that they now want to feel different. Yet others may achieve these changes in degrees. But usually, when some awareness has been reached that something has been changed, the person is aware of it and acknowledges it.

At some stage in most people's bereavement process comes the question whether to move house or in other ways adjust to different living conditions. Widowed people may find that they are in too big a house. People who have been disabled may need different accommodation. Some people may want to live nearer to old friends or families. Such decisions are never easy, and should certainly not be taken quickly. Perhaps people who have moved here from other countries may want to return to their home country after a spouse dies. Nurses and other helpers may be asked by people what they should do in this regard. Helpers and counsellors cannot take the decision for a person, but may need to work through the decision-making process with someone.

The point at which some break is made may be a very important milestone in the life of a bereaved person. The goal may have been achieved, and it will often happen more unexpectedly than envisaged, and perhaps also more painlessly than anticipated. When such moments happen they have to be marked. It is a truism that unless we mark an event, the event will not mark us. The – or *a* – goal may have been reached, but now we need to celebrate it. This is often done in some symbolic way.

Rites of passage

Rituals are very important around the death of a person. But also in relation to losing health, objects or ideals. Many people identify rituals with religion, and perhaps not unjustly so. Rituals have symbolic meaning, trying, by their actions, to unite the seen and the unseen, the here and the hereafter, the material and the spiritual.

Most religions have their rituals concerning burial. The Christian churches have become much more sensitive to the needs of individuals and families as regards funerals, and services can often be created by people themselves, and do not have to follow some set pattern. It is very likely that clergy will also create services for purposes other than funerals, and they may be willing to mark special anniversaries or events with some rite or blessing.

The saying 'goodbye' which is such an important step for bereaved people may, however, not necessarily take place in any conventional way. Anna planted a couple of fuchsia bushes for Benjy. Other people plant trees, or buy park benches. These are important actions and gestures. But they do not necessarily indicate that the bereaved person has reached a particular stage or point of detachment. The 'rites of passage' which are necessary for that may be very individual.

Ward and Wild (1995, pp. 108–9) describe a woman who had recently separated from her husband and left the marital home. She went back to it on a day when she knew that her ex-husband would be away. She cleaned the house from top to bottom, cut flowers from the garden and put them in every vase she could find, played her favourite music, and finally had a bath and changed her clothing. In this way she said 'goodbye' to her marriage, home, and the life she had there.

Stone (1980) describes a

funeral which was more of an actual farewell than the original burial. It was the placing, by a widower, in a specially dug ditch in the garden, of all the personal clothing which had once belonged to his long-dead wife. After his private ceremony he told friends that 'he felt lighter'.

Another 'burial' which I found very moving was an inspired rite de passage given by friends moving from a too large country house. The house was now too large because family had grown up and moved away. In a huge bonfire in the garden was stacked all the old unwanted furniture, and burnt at a party for generations of family and friends. Because this marked a symbolic death of family, there were tears among the laughter.

Many religions have special ceremonies to mark anniversaries of deaths and burial and it can be very helpful for people to follow these. Where there are no religious ties, people will often mark the site of a tragedy or event with flowers, even years later. Decorating the graves of families and friends is an important activity. It is said that in one cemetery in London, which has large underground catacombs, the bereaved used to come every Saturday morning, when the doors were opened, and bring their picnics and needlework. This is similar to the feasting which happens in cemeteries in Muslim societies on certain festivals.

Rituals of a corporate and private kind give people a legitimate form of expression for their feelings. It is often not possible, though, to do anything spectacular or even special for some people. Writing a poem, painting a picture, working an embroidery, or perhaps *not* making Christmas puddings (see Chapter 4) are nevertheless also important ways of marking the ending of something which was important.

In counselling it is also possible to use techniques like 'the empty chair' to help people to say something to the person (who is figuratively sitting on the chair) which still needs to be said; or by using visualization to encounter a person and in this way to help the bereaved to disengage. Such techniques do not need much training, but they should not be done by people who have not experienced them themselves. Even then, there needs to be some knowledge of such processes, in particular how to bring people back again into the here and now.

This chapter started with the loss of pets and ends with rites and rituals, which may seem a little odd. But it is not the subject itself which matters so much when considering how to help bereaved people. People who have lost something or someone important have the loss in common; helping them is therefore very similar, even if the circumstances differ widely.

Further reading   Lee, L. & Lee, M. (1992) *Absent Friend: Coping With the Loss of a Treasured Pet.* High Wycombe: Henston.

Mulrain, G. (1995) Bereavement counselling among African Caribbean people in Britain. *Contact; The Interdisciplinary Journal of Pastoral Studies* **118**: 9–14.

CHAPTER TWELVE

Loss of youth and independence
Challenging

....

Muriel was just gone 60. She had been severely spastic (her expression) from birth and had some difficulty in talking. Despite this she had managed an independent life. She had, however, never been to a school, but was educated at home, and she had never considered that she might have a job. She had long ago had all her teeth removed and wore dentures. Her eyesight had begun to deteriorate seriously when she was 50, and she needed frequent changes of spectacles. Her hair, which had always been lovely and naturally curly, had begun to fall out for no apparent reason and she had to buy a wig.

She had to move out of the house in which she was living because it was due to be demolished. So she came to live in sheltered housing where she was also provided with various kinds of help. A bath attendant came twice a week, and she gradually heard Muriel's story.

Muriel had never married, and this was beginning to weigh on her mind. In fact she described how, when she was a young adult, her mother shielded her so much that she was never with young men. One day now she said with anger and disappointment in her voice, that she had never seen a naked man. She often longed for intimacy but did not know what it might involve. She could identify feelings of sexual desires, but it was the bath attendant who one day told her about self-pleasuring; Muriel had not known about it. She trusted her bath attendant enough to ask her to show her what this might mean, but the bath attendant politely declined, knowing that this could be against her regulations. She pointed this out to Muriel, who accepted to be given verbal explanations.

Over a period of about two years, Muriel became steadily more dependent: she needed an electric wheelchair to get about; she needed meals on wheels, and instead of going on holidays, as she had often done, she needed to be content with people visiting her at their con-

venience. One day she fell out of her wheelchair and broke the head of her femur. She was much stiffer after that and needed help with dressing. Most of all, she became very slow, and this meant in particular that she could not get dressed in time to go to church on Sundays, which had been her practice all her life. She found this very depressing.

She often resented this slide into dependence when she already had an unequal start in life. Her bath attendant was a woman of younger years, but they formed a close friendship, and Muriel saw this as the one bonus of her present life.

Gerry had found the years between 40 and 50 to be immensely difficult. He had a good job and a loving family, but something was still missing in his life and he could not put his finger onto it.

The children were taller than him, and he had stopped competing with them at games. One child had got married and Gerry had become a grandfather. Instead of being proud to 'give his daughter away' at the wedding, it had propelled him into a depression which lasted several weeks. He did not want to give his daughter away, but wanted to keep her – somehow as a reminder of his manly vigour. The arrival of the grandchild was another realization that he was over the hill.

He felt these things deeply, but managed to get on with life regardless. His wife often begged him to go to his doctor for help, but he was against taking pills, which is what he expected would happen.

His physique changed during this time, and he grew rounder and balder. He broke three teeth in a row, being reminded that elephants die when they cannot eat any longer because their teeth have fallen out.

Gerry knew exactly that this was his mid-life crisis, but even to admit this was abhorrent. He was not the sort of man to be soppy about such things.

One day he was cutting the hedge in his garden with an electric hedge trimmer and he let it drop, giving him a nasty cut in his right foot. He had to go to A&E and later visit his GP practice twice. He jokingly remarked to the nurse that he was now even too weak to hold an electric hedge trimmer. She noticed some irony in his voice when he said this and asked him what this meant for him. Ten minutes later Gerry left, with an appointment to see the counsellor at the practice. He never thought that he would need 'a mini-shrink', but the six times which he went there, he admitted, should have been provided also when he was 20, and 30, and 40.

Loss of youth

'You are old, Father William', the young man said,
'And your hair has become very white;

And yet you incessantly stand on your head -
Do you think, at your age, it is right?'
(Lewis Carrol, *Alice's Adventures in Wonderland*)

The young cannot understand the old, and the old would like to be still like the young – at least this is the stereotypical image. Our culture is one in which youth is exalted and old age often dismissed. But this may be changing. The growing number of elderly and old people will not and cannot be forgotten.

This chapter deals with losses which happen gradually for the most part, and are perceptions as much as facts. There is seldom a clear point when someone declares having lost youth or vigour. Many people, when asked if they feel their age, will say that in their heart they feel as young as ever. It is only their body which is growing old. The age one feels, however, is not necessarily tied to a figure – 20 or 30 – but more to an image of oneself as a person who is capable of functioning adequately for the tasks in hand and requested.

'Growing old gracefully' is perhaps something which most people would like to happen or be said of themselves. This means, adjusting to the ageing process without too much ill health and certainly without too much exhibition of regrets, and bitterness. Quite how one adjusts to getting older and old age is however not something which one learns in a course or at school. Workshops and seminars exploring living in the second half of life are popular in some circles, but it may be that people who go to such events are those who have the inner resources already.

Young people find it difficult to imagine what life might be like when they are older, and older people find it frequently quite difficult to take orders from people who are younger than themselves. A shift in perception has to come in at some stage which accepts that the younger people are just as capable and knowledgable. At the same time there also has to be a shift into the role of 'elder' and perhaps expert, leader or person who is looked up to and admired. Later still, that role too, may have to be relinquished again.

There are so many negative stereotypes around the issue of getting older and old age that many people dread getting old. The search for the elixir of youth is also very ancient, and every age has had its means of keeping young and defying age and death. It is this fear of death which old age brings with itself, which had no doubt been the driving force behind the desire to stay young. When one admits to old age, one admits to decline, going downhill and having one foot in the grave. Perhaps the association with death makes younger people shun older ones.

The diminishing of health and physical vigour is usually so gradual that it is not noticed. When does one's skin begin to wrinkle? When does the voice change? The first grey hair may be noticed, but when this happens at 30, it is dismissed as freakish. When all of a sudden a few teeth break, it is considered more like bad luck than a definite sign of old age. It is perhaps not until someone makes a remark about one's age, or a health check reveals certain unwanted signs, that one becomes aware of age. Or perhaps it is that others notice certain mental capacities failing, such as memory. Or, as someone once said, old age is the time when the slim waist and broad mind change places. The hardening of the arteries can also lead to a hardening of views and opinions.

The slide into greater dependence is also imperceptible. But many people fear – or rail against – having to use cups with two handles again, wear incontinence pads which look like nappies, and literally in the evening take off their wig, their hearing aid, their spectacles, their dentures, and put on their splints, vests and bandages. Is it any wonder that Shakespeare talks of 'second childishness'?

Against this, Johnstone (1991) writes:

my father-in-law, who is a psychotherapist, once told me of a feeling he sometimes had about senility. Perhaps, he wondered, the apparently aimless wanderings in time which the young find so confusing in the old, are really a sort of journey from place to place in memory, spinning a chrysalis to contain their real shapes ready to leave this world like spaceships to a distant star.

Loss of mental function

Age and ageing often brings with it not only the loss of physical ability, but also of mental ability. This is not merely a slowing down of mental capacity or a loss of memory, but mental illnesses are more common in the elderly. Dementia, Alzheimer's Disease and depression 'affect a comparatively small number of older adults' (Schofield, 1995, p. 142), but they cannot be disregarded. According to Schofield, dementia is the most frequent form of mental illness in the elderly, affecting 7% of the population over 65 and 20% over 80. One aspect of ageism is to present all older people as slow, half-witted and depressed.

Riggans (1992) writes that:

as a sister with responsibility for clinical care in a psychogeriatric assessment unit, I am convinced that the effects of loss and bereavement lie at the heart of many of the mental health problems experienced by elderly people and their relatives.

Since most people with dementia are cared for at home, their carers suffer with them, but often in a different way. Riggans writes of a daughter who was grieving the loss of her father's personality, and says that '(l)osing [the] loved one's personality is just as traumatic as any other type of loss. But because the loved one is still alive, few carers are aware of what is happening to them'.

When nurses and health carers come in contact with older patients and clients who are suffering from mental health problems, perhaps they need to be just as aware of the needs of their carers as of the persons themselves.

Accepting the loss of youth

Payne (1994) writes movingly about his realization of a new phase of his life.

I found the most powerful experience crossing out my mother's name against the 'next of kin' entry in my diary, and writing in my son's name instead. It was an unmistakable symbol of the passing of a generation, the transfer of power and responsibility within a family.

Perhaps most of us find it possible to adjust to our ageing physique. What is less easy to accept is the emotional side-lining which often goes with becoming older. 'Am I invisible? Have I lost my right to respect and dignity? What would happen if the roles were reversed? I am still a human being. I would like to be treated as one' (Seaver, 1994), writes a woman living in a nursing home. She writes of a fellow-resident who died on the day she wrote. 'He was a loner who at one time started a business and developed a multimillion-dollar company. His children moved him here when he could no longer control his bowels'. It is easy to feel that it takes little before we are put on the scrap heap. If we put ourselves there, that is one thing, but being put there by people who decide for us is quite another. The loss of control over life and living which so often goes with being ill or elderly is one of the biggest factors which can make a life intolerable and useless. Losing some body functions and capacities does not mean that people should lose their rights at the same time. The battle against ageism is concentrated in this area.

We need to be able to accept that youth is lost, but this should not make us victims in and of old age.

Another area which is often keenly experienced as loss of youth is when a woman reaches the menopause. Not only is the reproductive possibility lost, but the changes which go on in the body are often perceived as making the person less attractive sexually. The menopause is often also a difficult time for women, when they feel physically unwell, often put on weight (but in the 'wrong' places) and are perhaps emotionally liable to mood swings. Such signs are visible reminders of the passing years. It then becomes almost impossible to have any further children, and for women who either could not have or for various reasons did not have children, this can be a severe strain (see Chapter 6). Particularly when people have lost children, reaching the menopause may mean that any hope of having further children disappears.

Some people are pleased to reach the menopause. Women certainly feel different once they have reached this point in life, but it depends from which point they view these changes. Certainly the health and cosmetic industry is making the most of the changes which women feel and give them every encouragement to look after their bodies. The transition from 'youth' to older age, or maturity, need not be seen as a loss, and can also be a gain.

It is not only women who experience changes around the middle of life. Men, too, often go through severe mid-life crises. It is impossible to say if the external circumstances affect the internal patterns, or the other way around, but often men decide in their fourth decade that they want to spend more time with their families, or change a career (see story of Harry, Chapter 2), or pursue an interest which had always been there but which had to be suppressed because of other pressures. It is often at this time that people who were described as shy lose their inhibitions and become forceful, or others who have always been leaders may decide that this is no longer what they want to do.

Many people are asked – or ask themselves – to retire early. This can sometimes happen before the age of 50. If chosen or not, the result is that people have a lot of time on their hands. This can be a bonus, but also a burden. As a society we put much emphasis on being productive, or equate being 'unproductive' with being burdensome.

The loss of youth can be a depressing realization, especially if people have no particular aim in life. Those who have always lived for their work often find that losing work means losing 'everything'. This means specially losing a purpose for living. People who perhaps tend to be of an introverted nature, or have less intellectual ability, may find such transitions extremely difficult.

At the time of mid-life often the first serious health problems begin to present themselves. People who may have been very healthy find that their bodies simply do not function as well as before. We have come to see our bodies in very mechanistic terms: put in the right things at the top and the whole machinery works well. But bodies are more subtle than this. They also wear out more subtly. And they cannot be taken to pieces like machines. But we have also learned to replace many of the malfunctioning parts, and 'spare part surgery' is one way of keeping fit and young. Perhaps this is what Dylan Thomas meant when he wrote,

Do not go gentle into that good night,
Old age should burn and rave at close of day;
Rage, rage against the dying of the light
('Do Not go Gentle into that Good Night', 1952).

But do people really want to stay young? This may be a question which cannot have a simple answer. People change, and with them change also their surroundings, views and possibilities. This means that what once may have been a disaster can come to be seen as a gift; and equally, what once may have been positive, now may turn negative and become destructive. It may therefore be important to consider what goals there are in life, and perhaps keep to them.

Prolonged grief

Since the assumption is that nurses and health care workers 'accidentally' come across patients and clients who are grieving for some loss, it is quite likely that they will meet people whose mourning is pathological.

The fact is that the mourned person, object or value fades from the memory simply by the passage of time. But the grief which this caused is maintained by various different methods. Worden (1991, pp. 75–7) lists a number of clues which should make therapists (and helpers) aware that a person is suffering from unresolved grief:

1) The person cannot speak about the deceased without experiencing deep and fresh grief.

2) Some relatively minor event triggers off an intense grief reaction (see Benjy the rabbit, Chapter 11).

3) Themes of loss come up in interviews (see Muriel, above).

4) The person is unwilling to move material possessions belonging to the deceased.

5) The person's medical records reveal that they developed physical symptoms like those the deceased experienced before death.

6) People may make radical changes in their life-style and exclude from their life friends and family members associated with the deceased.

7) A person may have a long history of subclinical depression, often marked by persistent guilt and lowered self-esteem (see story of Robert and Sheila, Chapter 8).

8) There may be a compulsion to imitate the dead person.

9) There may be self-destructive impulses present (see story of Gareth, Chapter 7).

10) Unaccountable sadness occurring at a certain time each year (see 'Christmas puddings', Chapter 4).

11) A phobia about illness or death related to the specific disease from which the person died, e.g. cancer.

12) Persons may avoid visiting the grave or participating in death-related rituals or activities.

Rando (1984) writes about unresolved grief in great detail, describing the forms it takes, symptoms and behaviours, reasons for it, and problems caused by social roles. When grief is prolonged it becomes clear that people will have had some predisposing factors before the loss, such as an inadequate ego development, an excessive dependency upon the deceased, multiple losses, or guilt from other factors which may now block out any possible adjustment. Sometimes diasters or there not being a body can also precipitate prolonged grief.

It is recognized that people who suffer from prolonged grief need skilled and perhaps professional help. When people such as nurses and health care workers meet patients and clients who so suffer, it may be best to refer them to an agency or person who may be more specifically skilled. This is not undervaluing the helpers, but valuing the mourner rightly. The person who 'discovers' such a situation will have played as important a role as the therapist. Acknowledging grief and loss is often the first step in a process of adjustment, and as so much else in the area of counselling, bringing it into the open and saying the unspeakable, can be the most important thing and will be the turning point.

Challenging: how are you going to do it?

The last in the series of counselling skills to be described is the skill of challenging. It is not simply a skill which is only appropriate at the end of helping, but needs to be used throughout the helping process.

The whole of the helping process is a challenge. The critical step, for the client, is the step between recognizing a problem or unused opportunity, and doing something about it. Egan (1994, p. 32) says that the difference is between 'what do you want?' and 'what do you really want?'. In the model of the four questions which I have outlined here, the question is 'how are you going to do it?'

This question is the only really closed and quite specific question among the four. It is not a question of further exploration, but a question which points at an action and to a commitment. This question will be considered practically within the framework of the loss of youth and independence. It is of course not restricted to this type of loss, but applies to all types of helping. This also applies to helping which is done on a long-term basis, but in particular it applies to short-term and perhaps one-off situations. It is in these settings that there has to be some practical outcome, otherwise they cannot be said to have helped.

The rites of passage described in Chapter 11 have an aspect of doing something about the change which is the source of the bereavement. But they do necessarily coincide with the mental or inner adaptations which have also to be made. It is much more difficult to change one's attitudes, but in order that this is possible, external changes have to be made, such as restoring a particular relationship, or going out again, or countering negative thoughts with positive ones.

Evans (1993) writes of her experience as a nurse on an oil-rig which exploded. She and her colleagues spent a night in a lifeboat where one of the men died. She blamed herself for his death by not being able to care for him adequately as she was too shocked. A friend and fellow nurse helped her by discussing with her the changes she had noticed in Evan's behaviour. She writes:

No one could know exactly what I went through and suffered that night in the lifeboat, but I was mistaken in the assumption that no one else could know and empathize with my pain, confusion and guilt. With my friend's help, I was able to escape what I believed was my own personal world of suffering. I was able to recognize the link between my feelings and my actions and begin to change my behaviour.

She does not say exactly what her actions were, but it is possible to guess that she interacted more freely again with colleagues because she did not need to carry the personal world of suffering like a burden all the time.

Rainey (1990) writes of a husband whose wife had become physically disabled. The husband's 'heartfelt loss was that he was unable to have a long conversation with his wife now because of her memory problems.' But then he discovered that reading to her in the evenings from the local paper helped them both to cope with their loss. The goal here may well have been to keep both people interested and responsive to each other, and one way of doing this was by this method of reading.

This may seem a small goal and a small achievement. But no goal is too small, and no achievement too insignificant. When people are traumatized they often have difficulties with tasks which seemed routine before, and with 'thinking straight' in relation to necessary tasks, therefore even such a seemingly simple way of implementing the goal is important.

This example also shows some other aspects of the helping process:

it shows that presumably the authors of the article and the couple had talked with each other;

that keeping interested and responsive to each other had been recognized as a need, even if the word 'goal' may never have been mentioned;

that perhaps the author had made some suggestions of how this goal might be achieved;

that perhaps she may have asked quite directly: 'how are you going to keep interested?' ('how are you going to do it?');

she may not have suggested reading the paper herself, but having been given a suggestion, perhaps the husband had come up with the idea himself;

that at some stage she may have asked the couple how they are getting on with reading the newspaper, and then it will have been seen that the husband could put into practice what he had seen as a goal.

The skill of challenging is an important one, but also one to use with care. It is not a confrontation like 'you have never managed this yet', but more like 'where do you see that you are going wrong?' Since it is the other person's goal which matters, not our own, it is the other person who has to make it work and who has to change in such a way that it can work. What helpers have to do is to challenge clients to be realistic with their goals, and also realistic in the way they want to pursue their goals.

When goals are too big or too high, they cannot be reached. At the first attempt to reach them, clients get despondent and disillusioned and this reinforces their helplessness. For this reason goals have to be realistic and tailor-made to the person. The means of reaching the goals have to match the goals, and this is perhaps where helpers need to challenge most. 'Can you do this?' 'How realistic is it to talk with this person?' 'Is this the only way of doing it?' 'You have tried this before, what makes it different this time?'

When we challenge someone we take on a role of devil's advocate. This may give us an air of being more clever, or ahead of the client. When the core conditions – unconditional positive regard, congruence and empathy – are present, this can be seen to diminish. Challenging then becomes empathy, because it is done from a position of sharing the client's aims. When we are able to feel at home in the client's perceptual world, we are using the language and expressions with which the client is familiar. It is only when we stand outside this world and are perhaps more concerned with our success or failure in a helping situation, that challenging can become judgemental. This is something which may always need to be kept in mind.

Anderson and Dimond (1995) and Garrett (1987) cite a number of coping strategies which bereaved people can adopt, such as learning new skills, learning to socialize as a single person, keeping busy, helping others, joining groups to pursue interests in hobbies, religious and recreational activities, keeping fit, and sustaining family ties. These are very practical ways of adapting to bereavement. It is often not the opportunities which lack, but the person's own willingness to give these possibilities a go. People who have been bereaved can at times live so much in their own world of suffering that they cannot bring themselves to leave it. With empathy helpers are able to enter that world, but also the know-how not to become absorbed in it. As helpers we need to keep our own world clearly in view. It is from within the perspective of our own world that we can offer challenges to the other person: not to then enter *our* world, or to imply that ours is the *real* world, but to create *their* own world around them which offers them health and wholeness.

The hope

The hope in any helping work surrounding loss and grief is that the person can adjust and live again. It will be a different life, but not a less valuable life. Most of us have a tendency to compare before and after, or one person with another. This is often not helpful, because no two people are the same, and life is not a competition. A loss, of whatever kind, is only a loss because we had some attachment to the person, object or value, and we mourn the pain of the loss. When we allow ourselves to feel the pain then we can also allow the pain to be healed.

The image of the 'wounded healer' is well-known in nursing and medical literature: those who have been wounded and healed can then heal others. But those who have not dared to be healed cannot heal others. To some extent we are all wounded and are all partially healed and partially suffering. It is not the completion which counts, but the effort towards completion. In the same way the hope which helpers (healers) convey to those whom they try to help is that life *can* be good again – if we dare. This is a challenge if ever there was one.

Further reading

Knight, B. (1986) *Psychotherapy with Older Adults*. London: Sage.

Scrutton, S. (1989) *Counselling Older People: A Creative Response to Ageing*. London: Edward Arnold.

CHAPTER THIRTEEN

Loss of beliefs and values
Beginning and sustaining relationships

....

Barbara's brother, Aidan, had been suffering from manic depression since his early adult life. It had become clear when he was at university that there were more problems than normal for people of his age and in his surroundings. Over the years he spent time in hospital, was a few times in prison, but was mostly at home. Their parents did everything to make his life as pleasant as possible and theirs not too impossible. They seemed to have endless patience and a capacity for tolerance which often left Barbara to marvel.

All said and done, the social service care which Aidan got was decent. But when first one and then the other parent died, Aidan became violent and needed hospital care again. He was there for over a year without apparently getting better. Then a psychiatrist decided that a new type of drug should be tried. Aidan responded very well and plans were made for his discharge. Since he had a home, everything was tried to get him back.

But nobody seemed to listen to Barbara who insisted that she could not look after him. He was much improved, everyone assured her, and he would be able to cope much better. He came home, and indeed seemed much improved. But at home he was alone, with Barbara working some distance away. Aidan, not unnaturally, went out most of the day. One evening he was not back as usual, and Barbara raised the alarm. Listening to the local news that evening she heard that a woman had been assaulted quite close to her home, but she had no reason to think that this has anything to do with Aidan. Not until the police rang. Aidan had assaulted the woman, jumping at her from behind a hedge, producing a kitchen knife which Barbara recognized. She was so badly injured that she died three days later. Aidan was arrested and held in custody.

When the story was pieced together, it appeared that patients on that particular drug needed regular check-ups and blood tests, but Aidan had not known about this. He had in fact been left without any supervision altogether.

Barbara was not only shocked by the event itself, but she was profoundly disillusioned by the treatment her brother received. As time wore on, she felt that she could not trust any medical staff any longer. She knew that the NHS was in a bad way, but this was beyond belief.

The tragedy affected her in other ways, too. From having been a practising Christian, she began to question her faith and beliefs. She found it difficult to reconcile what was happening to her with what she heard in church. She seemed to have been abandoned by her family, by social services, and by God. At one time there seemed to have been love and care, but this tragedy had robbed her of the possibility to believe in the goodness of either God or people. What was more, no-one at the church seemed to have noticed that she did not attend there any more. This reinforced her disillusionment. The loss of her faith, her beliefs and her reasons for them, caused her such pain that she finally sought refuge in alcohol. At least this would drown her sorrows for a while. It was not until she lost her job that a personnel manager helped her to get in touch with Alcoholics Anonymous.

Some of the people mentioned in earlier stories either made the following remarks or implied them.

There is no point in living any longer; I am tired of life (Donald, Chapter 2).

I can't forgive that man for being careless. He has destroyed my life (Susan, Chapter 3).

I have done the worst. I could never face people again (Alex, Chapter 4).

I have lost hope (Terry, Chapter 5).

I have lost belief in myself (Gareth, Chapter 7).

I will always have to pay for my mistakes (Sheila, Chapter 8).

I cannot trust politicians. Now I know that all people are racists (Kingsley, Chapter 9).

I am in danger of never again becoming attached to things (The Caravan, Chapter 10).

I cannot trust adults (Anna, Chapter 11).

I have lost self-respect (Gerry, Chapter 12).

I have lost faith (Barbara, above).

Loss of beliefs and values

This chapter deals with the more intangible aspects of loss – those, in fact, which we may be loathe to admit. They may be very personal experiences, and many times we may not be consciously aware of 'having' these beliefs and 'holding' any particular tenet because they are intrinsic parts of ourselves. Not until we come up against some situation where they are either questioned or we as a person are confronted with them, do we perhaps know that now they are gone.

Some of the beliefs and values described in this chapter have been mentioned before, some overlap each other, and some may mean very similar things. And they are by no means all such values which could be mentioned.

By describing the *loss* of the values and beliefs, this may only be one side of the experience. Some people might simply consider what is happening as a stage in life and a transition to other and presumably better values. The point is, as with so many of the other aspects of loss described, if a person experiences something as loss, it is a loss to that person. Perhaps with the help which we can provide, the person might come to see that there might be other (and perhaps better) ways of viewing a situation. But in the first instance we need to hear the story and acknowledge the loss.

Loss of faith

We all have faith in certain things. We have faith in God, people, ourselves, to be and do certain things. This is based more on implicit trust rather than evidence. Faith often has to do with reciprocity: if we keep faith with God, God will keep faith with us; if we trust a certain person or process, that person or process will trust us and perhaps reward us.

When we lose such faith, we may feel that nothing and nobody can be relied on any longer. We are in the world by ourselves. If we want anything, we need to get it ourselves. This tends to make people self-reliant and perhaps ruthless in getting always what they want. Therefore losing faith could imply that people have not only lost something, but have had to acquire something – go-getting and egoism – which they did not like in others and certainly do not like in themselves. But, they complain, 'they' pushed them towards such a stance. There may therefore be a resignation about such a person which can border on the hopeless.

Loss of belief

Faith and belief have much in common. Belief may imply something more concrete, perhaps asserting a creed or a set of dogmas. Campell (1987, p. 89) makes a distinction between 'the act of faith = the faith by which one believes, and the content of faith = the faith which is believed'. But this seems not to be all there is to faith; faith is essentially about trust, and therefore losing faith is often equated with losing trust.

The loosening of patterns of authority has led many people to change their beliefs. In a world where there is cohesion between beliefs and actions, everyone is expected to follow the norm. This is perhaps the image many people have of life in the past and they yearn to have certainties again. Because these have gone, and we have moved more or less strongly with the tide, our own certainties have disappeared.

It is possible to blame this or that person or cause for the loss of belief – be this religious belief or belief in particular values – and mourn this loss. The loss of religious belief can be very painful, perhaps excluding a person from participation in life-styles and practices which had shaped life hitherto. Such loss may also lead to shame: 'what will people think of me?'. It may be a loss which may not be easily or openly admitted, but felt deeply and perhaps leading to desperation and intense loneliness.

Loss of certainties

We all have different certainties. Like beliefs and faith, they give a stability and backbone to our lives which make it possible to keep on living.

The certainties which people have are built on some experience: the love of parents or a partner is certain. The houses which we live in are safe. As long as we are healthy, we can also be certain that tomorrow we will wake up again feeling not much different from today. Benjamin Franklin said that 'in this world nothing can be said to be certain except death and taxes'.

Many other things are less certain. We can never be completely certain that a particular train will run, or that a certain machine will work. We cannot rely on friends to support us in every instance.

Perhaps the assurance of a partner's love is the most unconditional certainty we have. When this trust is broken, then something vital has been lost. This can be such a drastic loss that the loss of this one certainty can cause the collapse of trust altogether. We can never again feel that we can really trust another person, let alone another person's assurance of love. When a person has lost that certainty and that trustfulness, there will no doubt be immense grief.

Loss of purpose

After the loss of a spouse, partner, job, pet, or any other significant person or object, there is often a concomitant loss of purpose. When the main object of love and admiration has gone, the person needs to readjust to life without that person or motivation for living. In the first days and weeks there may be a severe disequilibrium. People may have cared for someone at home for months and years, and when that person dies, there is nothing more for them to do. The purpose of their living has gone into the grave with the deceased.

This loss of purpose can lead to depression and personal neglect. While it is understandable, those who are around bereaved people may need to help them particularly to refocus their lives and find a new meaning and purpose for living. Sometimes this is not easy, and helpers should not imagine that they can 'snap' people out of such states. They need support and attention, not platitudes.

Loss of values

What are today usually known as values might have been described as virtues in the past. When we say that we value certain people, we probably mean that we admire their courage, trustfulness, reliability, friendship, honesty, etc. When we value a certain service, we probably mean that we can rely on it, that it is good, does no harm, promotes certain views which correspond to ours, etc.

When we say that we have lost certain values we may mean that we cannot trust others any longer for certain reasons; we used to be honest but found that it did not help and therefore had to start being dishonest 'like everybody else'; we thought that thrift was a way of life, but then found that nobody else thought that this was a good thing. When we suddenly wake up to some facts, we become disillusioned with 'the world', 'them', ourselves, society. This can be a severe blow to some

people. The thought that we were trying to live in and con-
struct a decent society, only to find that all our work and
attempts to be good citizens were to no avail and even being
ridiculed, may make some people very bitter. Losing the
values which we had been taught by our 'elders and betters'
may also mean that we let *them* down, not just ourselves.
When such a realization comes over somebody, there may be
a deep sense of loss and bereavement.

It is not only old, or older, people who experience a sense
of loss of values; many young people go through the same
process, particularly when first going to live away from home.

Perhaps it is a sign of the times that in ethical debates the
notion of 'virtue' is gaining acceptance again. In nursing, too, the
idea of 'virtue ethics' is being strongly advocated (Scott, 1995).

Loss of traditions

This may be an area which is particularly experienced by
people going to live in other cultures and societies. Minority
groups of people of any description may find that when they
move out of their own traditions that they cannot behave, celebrate and live in ways which had been meaningful to them.
This goes for families as well as groups and societies of
people.

The loss of traditions is often associated with cultural and
religious expressions. Where there was a cohesion once, for
various reasons this is lost. The surrounding culture may not
easily tolerate differences, forcing people to behave like
'them' in order to be accepted. If this does not happen, there
may be harassment on both sides. Wanting, or needing, to
conform always leads to a loss of distinctiveness. This can be
felt very keenly by those who have to do the adapting. It may
be felt more as anger than sadness: it is an anger against the
hardness and stubbornness of the surrounding culture. The
fact that often the two cultures or societies cannot speak each
other's language makes the gap even wider. If they could talk
with each other and hear each other's stories, there may be
more opportunity to remain oneself and not lose the very
things which matter most.

Loss of norms

By loss of norms may here be thought certain ways of behaving, like queuing for services, or saying 'please' or 'thank you',

giving up one's seat for an older person, or other details of etiquette. These were ways of life which were highly regarded in an earlier society, but losing them makes many people aware that they live now in a different age. This can be painful. Having been brought up to be a 'decent' person, but finding that other people are not in the same way interested in keeping up with certain standards, makes some people feel very different and even outcast. The British enjoy a certain eccentricity, and rather than be despondent about being different, some people 'take on' the world and stick to norms which may now be either in decline or not valued any longer.

Loss of self-respect

When some of the elements described here are lost, there is a further loss: that of self-respect. 'Who am I now that this has happened?' It becomes difficult to believe in ourselves. We know ourselves as one kind of person, but something has changed us, and we no longer recognize who or what we are. As such we may act in a particular way which is actually abhorrent to us. We cannot trust other people any longer – but now we cannot trust ourselves any longer.

Self-doubt is a common experience of many people, but there comes a point when we feel we are not worth anything and not worthy to be here. The guilt which many people experience after the death of a loved person is closely allied to this way of thinking. For many people in this state there seems only one logical solution, which is suicide.

For elderly people this often means that they feel a burden and have nothing further to contribute to life. Therefore they would rather be dead. They may ask to be put out of their misery.

This kind of despair has to be taken seriously. Most people have more will to live, even in difficult circumstances, than they often admit. The wish for oblivion may come from a deep hurt which may never have surfaced because the person may have been too ashamed or too shy to admit to it. A sensitive person, willing to hear what may turn out to be a 'confession', may help a person to a new understanding of an old hurt. The wish for death may not entirely disappear, but the living until death may become a great deal easier.

Loss of confidence

Many people find that after a big shock or loss they lose self-confidence. They find it difficult to concentrate, make decisions, or think clearly. Therefore they lose confidence. This does not normally last very long, but while it does last it can be a source of distress to someone. Someone who will always have acted confidently, and all of a sudden cannot, may wonder if she or he is going mad. This is often the conclusion from such a time – or at least the worry. When it can be pointed out to bereaved people that this is a normal reaction to shock, then it can be seen in context and perhaps be coped with more easily.

Loss of hope

Loss of beliefs, values, purpose and respect can easily lead to loss of hope. The despair which some people experience is very real and indicates that they see no reason for anything any longer. Even the knowledge that tomorrow they might wake up again can be a burden. Perhaps loss of hope is the ultimate loss.

Like all the other losses, this too must be taken seriously. We have the phrase 'while there is life there is hope'. This often means that people believe against all odds that a seriously ill person might get better. Once they give up this hope they also give up any struggle. This can be a move into reality. But it can also be a move in the opposite direction. When hope is gone, everything is gone.

Hope is not some cheap optimism, but for most people it is allied to a faith which keeps them going. It is therefore important to see what the person herself or himself understands by hope or faith, or any other belief and value. The empathy which comes with unconditional positive regard is perhaps alone able to get close to a person who has lost hope. It may take a lot of congruence on the part of a helper to be allowed into the 'inner world' of such a person, but once trust has been established, then there is also some hope, whatever it is, and however intangible and fragile.

Beginning and sustaining relationships

It could be said that the discussion about the helping relationship should have come right at the beginning of the book.

But the same might be said about everything else: everything in helping is so important that it should have priority.

A relationship exists between the helper and the helped if the interaction lasts just a few minutes or if there is on-going and long-term therapeutic work being done. In a short interaction the relationship may not be so significant, but it can never be under-rated. Someone who listens to another's story gives something significant to that other. Someone who can tell, perhaps even to a relative stranger, something important, gives that something because there is some trust. This matters enormously. Bayne *et al.* (1994, p. 31) write that 'Rogers argued that the relationship that develops between counsellor and client is the most significant agent of change, not the counsellor's repertoire of techniques'.

The first 'what is happening?' sends a signal of concern and empathy. Egan (1994, p. 117) says that in 'interpersonal communication, empathy is a tool of civility. Making an effort to get in touch with another's frame of reference sends a message of respect. Therefore, empathy plays an important part in building a working alliance with clients'.

It is sometimes said that helpers have to be one step ahead of clients in order to help realistically. This is perhaps not quite right. Helpers do not have to be more clever, knowledgeable or accomplished at solving problems. They do not have to be ahead. What they need is a certain objectivity, which permits them to enter the other person's personal space and to withdraw again without damaging themselves or the other. This is perhaps the most important contributions which helpers can make. Therefore they can enter into a relationship, as fully as is necessary, and withdraw also when the time comes. In a way they are therefore mirroring what the client also has to be able to do with grieving: the time for commitment to and sharing of the other's world has ended with the death of the loved one. Therefore a kind of stepping back into one's own world again is now necessary, in order to move on and engage with other people and relationships. This does not deny the total commitment made earlier, but because there is no longer the same commitment needed now, an adjustment has to be made. Such an understanding of the helping role makes the helper not better, but a partner; the two people share something.

Egan (1994, p. 60) describes helping as a 'process of social influence' because it is unilateral in nature. The helper is in a position of power over a person who is weaker. The way in which this power is used, therefore, is crucial. This is why

Rogers insisted so much on the core conditions of unconditional positive regard, congruence and empathy. Perhaps the
way in which we use our power at all levels, not only in helping, describes most specifically who and what we are as persons.

It has been said that one aim of helping is to empower
clients. If this means giving them power, then this may not
always be successful. Rather, it means helping the other person to use the power which he or she has already. But more
still, it means helping clients to discover in themselves the
powers which they have perhaps not dared to see or were
simply not aware existed. One of the main aims of many helping situations is to help clients to find their blind spots, consider their reasons, and then deal with them. It is not up to
helpers to say 'you are awfully blind about your capacities'
without very good reason. Said in the right circumstances and
with the right preparation and support, this may be a valid
challenging statement. But the helper will need to have 'ear-
ned' the right to make such a statement. The relationship will
need to be solidly trusting.

Every relationship begins with some introduction. This may
be no more than making eye contact. This is often enough
for people to make the other contacts which are necessary,
based more on subjectivity than objectivity. Most of us know
instinctively when we can trust a person simply by looking at
him or her, without knowing anything more about the person.
This is often the case in health care settings. Patients and
clients have little choice of their nurses and other care workers. The relationships which they therefore make with each
other is all the more important. It is clear that we cannot have
the same deep and firm relationships with everyone, but there
are usually one or two people to whom we feel particularly
close, and whom we can trust.

We can never impose ourselves on anyone. Just because we
may be in a position of power or help may not make us necessarily the ideal person to help everyone. But when we have
gained someone's trust, we have a professional obligation not
to destroy this.

When patients and clients tell us their very personal or intimate stories, we must be aware of confidentiality. Sometimes
we may hear of matters which may be crucial for better care,
but we can never assume that patients therefore want us to
tell the whole team. If we have gained a person's respect, this
means that the empathy which allowed the story to be told
also has to be a 'tool of civility' and means that we ask per-

mission, or at least share our intentions. Helping can only happen when we are aware of 'what you say after you said hello'. As helpers we have easy access to patients and often their secrets, too, but it matters how we sustain the relationship in which these are dealt with.

Relating to people who have lost beliefs and values

The relationship is important in all types of helping, not just in situations of loss, and then not just when beliefs and values have been lost. Like all the other sections of this book, this one, too, must be understood in relation to all others.

When people say that they have lost faith, or values, they are saying something about themselves which comes from the deepest (or highest) part of themselves. We can lose people and things, but when we lose the sense of ourselves, our reason for living and existing, we are touching on the core.

We can go for long stretches of life without ever really considering what we are living for, or what our aim in life is. It is only when we are challenged, for whatever reason, that we are confronted with such questions. And then we may perceive that we have lost, rather than gained, something. People who say that they have lost faith in something or someone, experience the different state mostly as one of loss. But other people may experience it as the opposite, and feel perhaps that old shackles have fallen away and they sense a freedom which was never there before.

The possibility is here that as helpers we meet a patient or client who, for some reason or another, says or admits to having lost something: health, a friend, a child, a partner, independence, or a sense of self. It is easy enough to tell strangers of the loss of something tangible. It gets progressively more difficult to admit to the loss of intangibles, such as confidence, or certainties. It may therefore only be after several meetings with a person that we may hear of such losses.

This means that a relationship has to be on-going. Many nurses and other health carers do have long-term relationships with patients, even if they may only be short encounters each time. It may be that such meetings are oriented only towards the practical needs, usually of a physical nature. In order that patients and their carers can explore feelings, they need time. And this is at a premium today.

It often does not need much time, and much can be achieved in a short time. The quality of the relationship is therefore very important. The way in which we say 'How are you?' matters: do we really want to know, or is it merely an opener

for 'all right'? Do we convey empathy, genuineness, warmth?
And how do we do that? Do we give the impression that we
are here just for this person, now? And that we are really interested?

We may be able to do it most of the time, but it is not
possible all the time; we are not super-human. But even then,
some form of 'civility' would ask of us to give perhaps a short
explanation why today there is no time or no opportunity.
Admitting that we are not in a position to listen may be more
helpful than simply not paying attention. Genuineness
demands that we are honest: we don't have to go to great
lengths in making excuses. A simple statement may be better.

But when we do have the time and opportunity to listen,
then we need to listen with the whole of ourselves. When we
do this, the clients can also talk with the whole of themselves.
This is when losses of various kinds can be talked about and
acknowledged. Sometimes just saying there is a loss helps a
person to feel better.

Losing deep beliefs and long-held values is often a blow.
When it happens we feel let down, and feel also that we let
others down. But we experience these aspects as loss only
because something else has come into view which has not
(yet) replaced the old certainty. We cannot cheer people up
with 'it isn't really that bad; you will probably feel better
tomorrow'. That, for someone who has been hurt, may wreck a
relationship altogether and be simply one more loss and hurt.

But helping people to see their losses of beliefs and values
in perspective is different. A loss is felt so keenly because
there has been a matching gain before. It is possible to see
that the basic patterns of life only exist because they are held
in a balance of opposites. We only appreciate light because
there is darkness. Health is only apparent because there is no
illness. In the same way it is possible to say that a loss of a
belief is only a loss because there was once a 'fullness'. The
task of the person who experiences the loss is not to regain
the loss, but by being aware of the loss, trying now to become
aware of the fullness again. Just as no two days are the same,
so no two opposite will ever be the same. In other words, the
fullness which is possible after the loss will be a different
fullness from the one which was lost. But that it is a fullness
is not in doubt if it is clear that the loss was a 'real' loss.
We all have different ways of experiencing this, but the basic
experience is similar for everyone. When we can see and
admit that the loss is not all there is to life, then there may
be a new perspective emerging. This may be the important

meaning or purpose which may present itself. As helpers we may put the idea of opposites to a person, but we cannot make them accept it. We may be able to help others to understand this concept, though.

A loss, of whatever kind, is not necessarily the last word. Life is such that it will go on with or without our contributions or feelings. But if we dare to go with life rather than against it, then we are truly human. This may take some help from those who are prepared to listen to fellow human beings.

Further reading Zohar, D. (1991) *The Quantum Self.* London: Flamingo.

CHAPTER FOURTEEN

Other losses
Ending relationships

....

Philippa had a very close relationship with Joseph, a man much older than her, and living abroad. He often came to stay with her, 'escaping' from the home where he lived. This was a home for retired professional people. Philippa was always happy to welcome Joseph, but they also agreed not to live permanently together. Joseph never told his family too much about his 'English family', and they never enquired too closely.

When Joseph came over for what turned out to be his last trip, he was severely incapacitated with a heart condition, but he promised to be back in three months. When Philippa therefore received a phone call from the home to say that Joseph had died in the night, she was as shocked as any spouse might be. She went to his funeral, which had been arranged by Joseph's family in line with their customs. At the funeral she knew that she was really the chief mourner, but the family largely ignored her.

Billy was an only child. His mother suffered from motor neurone disease which had gradually got worse but was not bad enough for her to need constant attention. His father worked a long distance away and came home rather late, leaving again early. So it fell on Billy to do much of the housework and the cooking.

The family had often discussed their situation. Billy's father wanted to keep his job because it was well paid and meant that they could afford help when it would be necessary. Billy agreed to do a good deal of housework. And his mother was a loving person, being concerned for their welfare. She did however have to go into hospital when Billy was 17 and she died when he was 18. It was not until then that he realized quite how much he had lost his childhood by having to care for his mother and essentially be responsible for the day-to-day running of the house. Then he began to resent his mother and increasingly hate her, which made his grieving difficult because of very conflicting emotions.

Other types of losses

There are so many types of losses possible that it would never do even to start to make a list of them. The important one would always be left out. But it is possible to consider some of them here.

Loss of friends

When someone dies, that person will probably have had some people who could be considered friends. These may have been life-long friends who had seen each other regularly or in any case had been in touch.

Some elderly people living alone will at least have counted a neighbour as a friend. Sometimes the friend is a hairdresser or a milkman. They may not have had much in common, but they will have seen each other and passed the time of day together. Sometimes one hears of elderly people who may hardly have managed in their own home, but when social services wanted to take them away into a home, the neighbours protested and spoke up for the person.

One may call someone a friend whom one sees at a club, a meeting of an interest group, or with whom one only speaks on business.

When such friends die, those who are left behind grieve just as much as anyone would. But they may grieve alone and perhaps misunderstood. Those around them may think and imply that it is not 'right' for someone to be upset unduly when 'only' a friend or acquaintance dies. After all, there was no blood relationship. Love – whatever this may mean to a person – is much more important than any conventional rules of kinship.

One can also count as friends those who have taught us in some way or another, even without knowing them. Most of us are influenced by writers, musicians or artists of many kinds, and when such people die we may be severely shaken and grieve.

Friends are often the forgotten people when it comes to dividing out the possessions someone may have left behind. A small memento would mean very much, but friends may not dare to ask for fear of being ridiculed.

Loss of secret lovers

The story of Philippa is one of thousands such stories. She and Joseph were not totally secret lovers, but they nevertheless did not have a relationship which could be openly acknowledged everywhere.

There is something mysterious and also exciting about secret relationships. Having secrets is almost part of asserting oneself. Having them in such a way that no-one else knows about them shows a kind of resourcefulness which is affirming.

Today's society has become more tolerant of unusual relationships in general, but when it comes to particular people, this may not be so easy to tolerate. We still like to keep to certain norms and being 'one of us' is still important, whatever we may say. Therefore having secret relationships and loves may not be admitted. When such a relationship ends, for whatever reason, one or both partners may feel very lonely and isolated in their grief. They may not find it easy to talk about it and this may possibly cause prolonged and perhaps abnormal griefs.

Loss of a gay partner

Homosexual relationships, like secret love, have become much more accepted generally. But what is general may not apply to the particular. Gay men and women do not necessarily come from milieux where this is the norm, but from settings where such relationships are frowned upon or condemned. Sometimes the realization that they are different can be as much of a shock to the person concerned as it may be to their families. 'Coming out' is often such a major step that this declaration alone can bring with it so much anger and hurt that the person concerned feels that he or she has only one option, and that is to move away.

Homosexual relationships are by their very definition different from heterosexual relationships. They may change more often, be more promiscuous, and be believed to be, if not in fact, more associated with the drug scene than heterosexual relationships.

Many gay people are surrounded by friends who are HIV positive and many friends may have died. This can be devastating, bringing them constantly in touch with loss, perhaps aware that they too may have to face an early death.

When a partner of a gay relationship dies, there can be enormous difficulties between families and the gay lover. When families have not known about the sexual orientation of a son or daughter, they may be shocked to find it out now. Gay

partners have been ousted from funerals and from having anything to do with arrangements of possessions and property.
When this happens on top of the loss of the person, the surviv-
ing partner loses doubly: the loved partner and the things
which might have helped him or her to feel some continuation
of the love.

Gay people have access to good bereavement and counselling services, and if necessary should be put in touch with
them, but this does not exclude help being given them when
necessary in any circumstances.

Loss of money

In a world where professional people have to be financially
smart, the loss of money from bad deals or bad creditors can
be devastating.

People have lost vast sums of money – sometimes their
life's savings – by trusting some business venture which then
collapsed. Through no fault of their own they find themselves
impoverished and perhaps at the mercy of the very people
they had tried to help. This has again and again happened to
elderly people, or those who had invested in pensions, where
a financial crash has left them penniless. This is a serious blow
and can be heartbreaking. Particularly when their whole
future is thereby put in jeopardy, losing their savings can
make people also lose faith in those whom they trusted.

Other people may lose money through gambling of various
kinds. This is a risk which they are essentially aware of, but
when it becomes a habit or an addiction, their reasoning powers may not always help them to cope with it. Families can
be ruined or destroyed through the indiscriminate use of
money. The person who gambles with money is often not the
one who suffers most, but those around him or her. They may
lose their livelihood and their respect, and this may influence
how they deal with any personal losses in the future.

Loss of time

All of us waste time, but when time is lost through other
people's carelessness, we tend to become resentful. We
become angry, and perhaps rightly so, and try to ensure that
it will not happen again. This may not be so easy.

Losing time by 'doing time' is another way of considering

this aspect. Again, this does not concern just the person who is imprisoned, but the families surrounding someone may feel acutely that their time has been curtailed too. Waiting for trials and verdicts, release from prison and detention, can mean that people's lives are put on hold; they cannot really live, but have all their efforts concentrated on a date or a statement. Being robbed of the time which thus passes may be felt very acutely.

There may also be the stigma which attaches itself to a person and his or her family which makes this whole situation that much more difficult. There may be multiple losses involved, particularly for the family, when someone is imprisoned.

Loss of rights

Prisoners lose many of their civil rights while they are detained, and this may be considered one way of punishing them. For people who may be unjustly imprisoned, this is even more of a blow because they may not have any possibility to defend themselves. Prisoners of conscience are in the most precarious situation, where they may not have any possibility of being heard.

Luckily, these are relatively unusual events, though still too frequent. What is much more common is that people in all walks of life have their rights curtailed.

When patients are not given enough information, or not the correct information, tests are not adequate (see Gareth, Chapter 7), when old people are treated as if they were children, when patients are coerced into operations, when people are put under pressure not to reveal certain activities – the list could go on – then they are deprived of their rights. This can have serious consequences. But most of all, it is a disrespect for the person concerned. It means that someone considers himself or herself better than someone else. This person caused someone else to lose something which may be vital.

We are all constantly in danger of losing our rights as people. We are also all guilty of having caused other people to lose their rights. In many subtle and not so subtle ways we use our power, perhaps only too late realizing what we might have done.

In such situations we have to ask the Four Questions not of the other, but of ourselves. 'What am I doing here?' 'What is the meaning of it?', that is, from what motive am I doing it? 'How can I change?' and 'What am I doing to change?'

The skills and core conditions mentioned so often are all intended to help other people, not to abuse them. It is perhaps empathy, which becomes 'a way of being', which can best guard against 'man's inhumanity to man'.

Loss of childhood

The story of Billy portrays the loss of his childhood by having to look after his handicapped mother. Billy had agreed all along to be involved with her care. But perhaps a child is not always able to make such a decision. Billy will have had no other points of reference with which to compare his situation. He had never known anything else. He may well have seen how his school mates had more time and more leisure, but as an only child he may not have been in a position, at least emotionally, to deny his mother what she needed. It was only when she died that he realized what normal living could mean, and then he became aware of what he had lost out on during all his years of growing up.

There are many ways of losing a childhood. Children who have lost one or both parents may feel that they have never possessed what should by rights be theirs.

Children who have been physically, sexually, materially, mentally, emotionally and spiritually abused have lost important parts of their childhood.

It is often only years later that such losses come to light, perhaps when relationships cannot be sustained, when they cannot sufficiently concentrate on work, or indeed, when another loss happens and the earlier, perhaps suppressed, loss of their innocence or dignity comes to the fore. The sense of loss of personality or personhood may make them angry and bitter against the perpetrators of such acts. Since they are often parents or relatives who also provide for the child in significant ways, it is very difficult to make sense of the emotional disarray often left behind. The loss experienced from abuse in early life is often far more significant than any other loss sustained later on.

When parents have a child in later life they may be very protective and perhaps not let the child be a child.

There are endless different ways of depriving a child of his or her childhood. This is often not realized until much later, and then the loss seems all the greater. If it had been realized at the time, it might have been corrected, or so one hopes. But then on top of the loss comes the realization that because one was not sufficiently assertive or forthright one may have lost many more years of happiness by harbouring guilt, pain and perhaps hate.

Loss of aspects of health

Chapter 7 dealt with loss of health in general, but here some particular aspects will be considered.

Women are very likely to feel a loss of femininity after a mastectomy; men may feel the loss of their masculinity after an operation for prostate enlargement or cancer.

The removal of a testis for cancer, which usually happens in younger men, has a similar effect.

People who have had colostomies raised often feel less sexually attractive, and may even fear to have sexual relations for fear of causing damage.

Some medications cause impotence in men and that can be a severe loss of their self-image.

People who may have been fighting against some illness for a very long time feel that they have used all their energies for this one cause, losing out on other aspects of living.

Losing sight or hearing is not only disabling, but can lead to severe depression stemming from the sense of loss at being deprived of aspects of normal life and living.

Mental illness may be a very severe loss in a person's life. The illness may make someone feel that she or he has lost years of life, living in a half-world or an unreal world. Mentally ill people may also keenly feel the loss of many of their human rights, such as making decisions for their own care.

The nurses' own loss

Last but by no means least in this overview, the losses which nurses and all health care workers suffer when a patient dies, must not be forgotten. This has been the cause of many debates: how best to handle the grief when a person dies whom we have nursed and looked after.

It is right that we get attached to people whom we nurse; we would not do our job properly otherwise. Most of us will remember some patients always, for many different reasons. When patients get better and go home, this is a vindication of our skills, but when patients die, it is not so much a criticism of our ability, as a loss of a person, someone who had given us something significant, a friendship, something which we shared.

All losses need to be mourned. The amount of the mourning and grieving varies with the loss. But unless we acknowledge the loss, the wound which is created in the psyche may
stay there and fester. When it is attended to, by talking about
it and sharing it with someone or a group of people, this can
be like a medicine for that burning and hurting wound. When
we pay attention to the pain, we are also more likely to get
better sooner.

As nurses we have a terrible reputation of helping other
people but not helping each other too well. If we want to be
really human, we always have to look after our own. 'Charity
begins at home'. This does not mean that we should *only* look
after ourselves; on the contrary, once we have looked after the
nearest and dearest, we can then better look after all the
others who need our attention.

Bereavement from disasters

Post-traumatic stress is now a well-known phenomenon.
People who were in a disaster, but not necessarily personally
affected, can also be severely shocked and bereaved. Hinks
(1991) wrote about his experience of being present at
Hillsborough when the disaster happened. He wrote that
initially he felt vulnerable and insecure, believing that he
might not cope if people made demands on him. His work as
a clinical nurse manager began to suffer. 'I *wanted* to change,
to feel different, to be more "normal", but somehow I couldn't
see when the turmoil would end'. It was not until a year after
the event that he sought help. When he began to meet with
other people who had also been there, and could share his
feelings with them, he began to put things into perspective.
'At Hillsborough 95 people died, 400 received hospital treatment and 730 were physically injured. But these statistics cannot tell the full story, There are many more who, like me,
witnessed the Hillsborough tragedy and are in need of counselling'.

The murder of Jamie Bulger affected the whole country in
one way or another. In the same way, the murder of head-
master Philip Lawrence will be long remembered. And in yet
another way, the name of Lockerbie will always be associated
with the bombing of an aircraft.

Disasters and tragedies happen every day. In every one of
them many people die, but many more are affected. Indeed,
the soul of a whole country will be touched. There is a time
of bereavement for everyone. When such disasters perhaps re-

open old wounds also, we may need to be especially careful and sensitive to each other's needs.

Ending relationships

People whose lives have been deeply affected by abuse, denial and destruction, may need long-term and professional help. Health care workers may not be sufficiently trained or qualified to give this. But what they can give, either as 'first aid' or to supplement therapy, is empathy, understanding and a listening ear.

The assumption throughout the book has been that nurses and health care workers meet patients and clients who may be experiencing pain and grief from some present loss, such as health, and in the course of discussion, both patient and helper may discover other losses experienced which may never have been completely resolved. When this happens it may be difficult for the client to know on which of the losses to concentrate. It may be useful for the helper at that stage to enquire which is uppermost in the patient's mind, or most important. Some people may feel embarrassed about feeling that an earlier loss is actually more important than the present one. We may have to assure clients that they need not be concerned. We may also have to 'warn' them that another day the other loss may be more important. One of the aspects of grieving is the fact that the scene can change very quickly. This is part of the mechanism of detachment.

Health care workers who use counselling skills may not have the luxury of working with someone in depth and over a period of time. They will therefore have to work more quickly, that is, be perhaps more specific about reaching some insight and goal, and enquire of the client how he or she is going to make the necessary changes. Such a helping intervention is more focused on action. When two people can meet for several times there may be more time and space to explore together in depth what the various losses mean and how they can be understood and dealt with. Whatever the possibility, it is important that the person of our concern is in a better place at the end than at the beginning. This is the aim of helping, and this must be kept in mind. Worden (1991, p. 87) has a warning at this stage:

(i)f the problem underlying the unresolved grief has been unexpressed anger, it is critical that once this anger has been identified and felt, the patient is helped to see that angry feelings do not preclude the positive feelings or vice versa. If the therapist merely evokes angry

feelings without seeing them adequately resolved, the patient may be worse off than before.

The story of Billy shows that anger developed in him after time, and because he was also very fond of his mother, this was a difficult issue. He may have needed some time to work through these feelings adequately. He may not have needed help constantly, but being made aware of his feelings, he will probably have needed some help to see that such conflicting feelings are all right and very legitimate.

It may be that in a one-off session there is neither the time nor the opportunity to evoke anger, but a patient may discuss with one nurse something and another nurse may pick up some other aspect later on and thus continue the work. This second nurse may then get the full rush of anger which may have been called up or developed in the meantime. The second nurse may not be aware of what went before in the way of help given, and may therefore have to ask very closely 'what is happening?' Each helper will each time have to ensure a satisfactory ending to a meeting.

Because of the nature of health care, many encounters with patients and clients are one-off and short. Even if there were a willingness for more in-depth work, there might not be the opportunity. Patient turn-over and staff shifts mean that it is almost unusual for a nurse and a patient – at least in hospital – to form really long-term relationships. Much more usual are the short encounters. When there is a long-term helping relationship which is fruitful, then the ending of that relationship may have to be planned carefully. Long or short, the relationship has to end on a positive note.

When people have some task in which to engage, the 'work' of helping goes on. Thus a short-term relationship can be as effective as any other because there is something to do as a result of meeting. Sometimes having a task is also long-term helping. Here it means that there is something to work on between sessions, meaning that the days or weeks in between are also focused and that the work does not only happen when the helper is present.

It is well known that people who mourn a loss and are helped by someone empathic will usually form a strong relationship with the helper. If the helper then leaves the relationship abruptly (for whatever reasons), the client will feel another loss and may deteriorate physically and emotionally. In order to avoid being ourselves the cause of more pain, we must be careful to end each meeting in a satisfactory way.

This does not mean that the client has changed from being in the depths to being on top of the world. It may at times mean that the person is more pensive and more searching, but that may be positive, particularly if a very important point has been reached and discussed. It may also mean that it is right, under the circumstances, to leave a patient to weep quietly. This may be what is needed. Or it may be necessary and right to leave a person without any words of ending being spoken. But this is only right if both people are aware of it being right. Otherwise it may be insensitivity and hardness on the part of the helper.

Ending the session may coincide with ending the relationship. Knowing when and how to end is as much a skill as is knowing when and how to say 'hello'. In the framework of the Four Questions, some indication from the client as to how he or she is going to do whatever needs to be done, is a very useful way of ending. This gives a positive orientation and commits the client to some action. What is spoken between two people has more weight than what may simply be thought and imagined.

In a one-off encounter there will not be any possibility for evaluation or for enquiry as to how the act of changing went. If the goal was realistic, and the 'how' also, then there is much more chance that it will be put into action. The helper has to trust the person, and this trust may be enough of an incentive to spur the client into action.

When evaluation is possible it will need to be of three elements:

1)   the person's own insights, goals and progress towards goals
2)   the kind of help given and the way in which it was given
3)   the relationship between helper and client.

The first element may be a simple enough review: how did the client get on with the tasks set and were the goals achieved? If not, there needs to be a consideration of what went wrong. The question 'what is happening?' needs to be asked again, and so the process may need to start again, perhaps in more depth, or perhaps in less – depending entirely on the situation. This should not necessarily be seen as failure, but as part of the process of adjusting and learning.

The analogy with some dance steps in triple time can be useful here. Two steps are taken forward, followed by one step back. The step back is necessary for the movement to go on. The 'step back' in the counselling situation may therefore also be necessary to reconsider perhaps a certain aspect of a goal or a task which had perhaps not worked as well as hoped.

Since counselling is about decisions for living and emotions to cope with living after loss, the above paragraph may seem very mechanistic. Living is not simply a series of well-defined movements or blocks which all fit into one another. What happens in a counselling session is much more fluid, but nevertheless, these elements do figure. But we may never need to use this sort of language to describe what happens. When we become skilled in helping others we learn to recognize the various changes which take place and we can respond to them adequately. What is said here is therefore only said to make helpers (and readers) aware that such movements do happen.

The second point which may have to be evaluated at the end of a helping relationship is how well, or otherwise, the helper functioned. This is not fishing for compliments. It can be very helpful for both parties to consider this question. What helped the client most? What helped least?

Finally, the relationship itself needs to be considered. How did the two people work together? Since most problems met in counselling are problems of relating and relationships – to oneself and to others – a look at how this relationship functioned is often necessary. This may not need to be done only at the end, but in fact often during the actual process of helping too. Helpers can sometimes challenge clients by considering how they function in the relationship with the counsellor and compare or draw parallels with relationships which they mention.

Sometimes, if there has been a long process of helping, the ending may have to be prepared well. Sometimes both people know when enough work has been done. But the ending should be talked about and considered and should be satisfactory for both. When this happens, then both will feel that the work which they had done together has made a difference to both their lives. We do not help others in order to be also helped ourselves, but when we help effectively, then we are indeed also helped ourselves.

Further reading

Lysons, K. (1978) *How to Cope with Hearing Loss.* London: Granada.

Shapiro, C.H. (1993) *When Part of the Self is Lost: Helping Clients Heal After Sexual and Reproductive Losses.* San Francisco, CA: Jossey-Bass.

Postscript

....

I am always wary of books with titles like 'the complete works of', or 'guide to'. Can something ever be complete?

As I reach the end of this book, I am more conscious of what I have left out than what I have covered. As I wrote, so many more aspects presented themselves.

I am conscious of not having addressed bereavement from the point of view of special people, such as people with learning disabilities; or societies, such as ethnic groups. I tell myself that there is not space for everything, but perhaps there should have been just for this ... or that ...

And have I written enough of the positive side of grief and mourning? The ways in which people can not only come through loss, but be stronger for it? Perhaps ...

You will have noticed by now that I like stories and analogies. So I will close with another story, or parable, which the author permitted me to use, hoping that it will say many of the things which I could not have said in the same evocative manner.

Once upon a time, twins were conceived. Seconds, minutes, hours passed as the two dormant lives developed. The spark of life glowed until it fanned fire with the formation of their embryonic brains. With their simple brains came feeling, and with feeling perception; a perception of surroundings, of each other, of self.

When they perceived the life of each other and their own life, they knew that life was good and they laughed and rejoiced, the one saying: 'lucky are we to have been conceived and to have this world' and the other chiming 'Blessed be the mother who gave us this life and each other'.

Each budded and grew arms and fingers, legs and toes. They churned and turned in their new-found world. They explored their world and in it found the cord which gave them life from the precious mother's blood. So they sang, 'How great is the love of the mother that she shares all she has with us'. And they were pleased and satisfied with their lot.

Weeks passed into months and with the advent of each new month they noticed a change in each other and each began to see change in himself. 'We are changing', said the one, 'What can it mean?' 'It means', replied the other, 'that we are drawing near to birth'. An unsettling chill crept over the two and they both feared, for they knew that birth meant leaving all their world behind. Said the one: 'Were it up to me, I would live here for ever'. 'We must be born', said the other. 'It has happened to all others who were here'. For indeed there was evidence of life there before as the mother had borne others.

'But mightn't there be a life after birth?' 'How can there be life after birth?' cried the one. 'Do we not shed our life cord and also the blood tissues? And have you ever talked to one that has been born? Has anyone ever re-entered the womb after birth? NO!' He fell into despair and in his despair he moaned, 'If the purpose of conception and all our growth is that it be ended in birth, then truly our life is absurd'.

Resigned to despair, the one stabbed the darkness with his unseeing eyes, and as he clutched his precious life cord to his chest said: 'If this is so, and life is absurd, then there really can be no mother'. 'But there is a mother', protested the other. 'Who else gave us nourishment and our world?' 'We get our own nourishment, and our world has always been here. And if there is a mother, where is she? Have you ever seen her? Does she ever talk to you? NO! We invented the mother because it satisfied a need in us. It made us feel secure and happy'.

Within a short time the twins, one surprised, the other with a relieved twinkle in his eyes, entered a new stage of life in the arms of their mother. (Wilson, 1995, pp. 144–5, reprinted with permission)

Appendix

....

Further reading

Bowlby, J. (1981) *Attachment and Loss*, Vol. 3: *Loss, Sadness and Depression*. Harmondsworth: Penguin.

Leick, N. & Davidsen-Nielsen, M. (1991) *Healing Pain: Attachment, Loss and Grief*. London: Tavistock and Routledge.

Marris, P. (1986) *Loss and Change*. London: Routledge and Kegan Paul.

Sherr, L. (1989) *Death, Dying, Bereavement and Loss: An Insight for Carers*. Oxford: Blackwell Scientific.

Ward, B. (1993) *Healing Grief: A Guide to Loss and Recovery*. London: Vermillion.

Ward, B. (1993) *Good Grief: Exploring Feelings, Loss and Death with Over Elevens and Adults*. London: Jessica Kingsley.

Wright, B. (1991) *Sudden Death: Intervention Skills for the Caring Professions*. Edinburgh: Churchill Livingstone.

Some useful addresses

Action for Victims of Medical Accidents
   1 London Road
   London SE23 3TP
   Tel: 0181 291 2793

Cruse
   Cruse House
   126 Sheen Road
   Richmond, Surrey
   TW9 1UR
   Tel: 0181 940 4818
   Bereavement Helpline: 0181 332 7227

SANDS (Stillbirth and Neonatal Death Society)
   28 Portland Place
   London W1 4DE

Tel: 0171 436 7940
Helpline: 0171 436 5881

Society of Compassionate Friends (for parents who have lost a child)
6 Denmark Street
Bristol BS1 5DQ
Tel: 0117 929 2778

There are many local charities and agencies which offer help for specific situations and needs. Consult local Yellow Pages, Thompson Directory, or call Citizens Advice Bureaux.

References

Anderson, K.L. & Dimond, M.F. (1995) The experience of bereavement in older adults. *Journal of Advanced Nursing* **22**: 308–315.

Anonymous (1993) A cry for help. *Nursing Times* **89** (4): 29–30.

Baro, F., Keirse, M. & Wouters, M. (1986) Spousal bereavement in the elderly. *Health Promotion* **1** (1): 35–48.

Bartley, M. & Fagin, L. (1990) Hospital admissions before and after shipyard closure. *British Journal of Psychiatry* **156**: 421–424.

Bayne, R., Horton, I., Merry, T. & Noyes, E. (1994) *The Counsellor's Handbook: A Practical A–Z Guide to Professional and Clinical Practice*. London: Chapman & Hall.

Blain, S. (1993) Attitudes to women undergoing TOP. *Nursing Standard* **7** (37): 30–33.

Bowlby, J. (1980) *Attachment and Loss*, Vol. 3, *Loss, Sadness and Depression*. Harmondsworth: Penguin.

Bowlby, J. & Parkes, C.M. (1970) Separation and loss. In: Anthony, E.J. & Koupernik, C. (eds) *International Yearbook for Child Psychiatry and Allied Disciplines*, Vol. 1, *The Child in His Family*. New York: John Wiley.

British Association for Counselling (1989) *Code of Ethics and Practice for Counselling Skills*. Rugby: BAC.

British Association for Counselling (1993) *Code of Ethics and Practice for Counsellors*. Rugby: BAC.

Bryan, E. (1992) Grieving for the loss of a twin at birth. *Professional Care of Mother and Child* **2** (9): 280–282.

Burnard, P. (1994) *Counselling Skills for Health Professionals* (2nd edn). London: Chapman & Hall.

Campbell A.V. (ed.) (1987) *Dictionary of Pastoral Care*. London: SPCK (Society for Promoting Christian Knowledge).

Carmack, B.J. (1991) Pet loss and the elderly. *Holistic Nursing Practice* **5** (2): 80–87.

Chapman, E.N. (1989) *Improving Relations at Work*. London: Kogan Page Ltd.

Chick, S. (1989) *I Never Told Her I Loved Her*. London: The Women's Press.

Clark, M.D. (1985) Loss of job status. *Nursing Times* **81** (1): 53–54.

Cohen, P. (1994) The loss adjusters. *Nursing Times* **90** (9): 14–15.

Coke, E. (1628) 'The Third Part of the Institutes of the Law of England' ch. 73: 162. Cited in *Oxford Dictionary of Quotations*, 1993, 4th edn, Oxford University Press.

Dalai Lama (1995) The man himself. Interview with Vanessa Baird. *The New Internationalist* No. 274: 26–27.

Davis, G. & Murch, M. (1992) Why do marriages break down? Reading 38, in Giddens, A. (ed.) *Human Societies: An Introductory Reader in Scoiology*. Cambridge: Polity Press, pp. 177–182.

Dominian, J. (1968) *Marital Breakdown*. Harmondsworth: Penguin.

Donne, John (1624) Devotions Upon Emergent Occasions 'Meditation XVII'. Cited in *Oxford Dictionary of Quotations* 4th edn, 1992, Oxford University Press.

Egan, G. (1990) *The Skilled Helper: A Systematic Approach to Effective Helping* (4th edn). Belmont, CA: Brooks/Cole.

Egan, G. (1994) *The Skilled Helper: A Systematic Approach to Effective Helping* (5th edn). Belmont, CA: Brooks/Cole.

Evans, J. (1993) Crisis, grief and loss. *Canadian Nurse/Infirmière Canadienne* **89** (8): 40–43.

Frankl, V. (1962) *Man's Search for Meaning; An Introduction to Logotherapy* (rev. edn). London: Hodder and Stoughton.

Garrett, J.E. (1987) Multiple losses in older adults. *Journal of Gerontological Nursing* **13** (8): 8–12.

Gass, K.A. & Chang, A.S. (1989) Appraisals of bereavement, coping, resources, and psychosocial health dysfunction in widows and widowers. *Nursing Research* **38** (1): 31–36.

Gibran, K. (1926) *The Prophet* (and 1980) London: Heinemann Ltd.

Gilchrist, A., Hannaford, P., Frank, P. *et al.* (1995) Termination of pregnancy and psychiatric morbity. *British Journal of Psychiatry* **167**: 243–248.

Gilligan, C. (1982) *In a Different Voice*. Cambridge, MA: Harvard University Press.

Gould, D. (1993) Women's health care. Chapter 17, in Hinchliff, S.M., Norman, S. & Schober, J.E. (eds) *Nursing Practice and Health Care* (2nd edn). London: Edward Arnold.

Harris, B.G., Sandelowski, M. & Holditch-Davis, D. (1991) Infertility ... and New Interpretations of Pregnancy Loss. *American Journal of Maternal/Child Nursing (MCN)* **16** (4): 217–220.

Heinzer, M.M. (1995) Loss of a parent in childhood: Attachment and coping in a model of adolescent resilience. *Holistic Nursing Practice* **9** (3): 27–37.

Hinks, M. (1991) You'll never walk alone. *Nursing Times* **87** (15): 34–35.

Holmes, T.H. & Rahe, R.H. (1967) The social adjustment rating scale. *Journal of Psychosomatic Research* **11**: 213–218.

Hull, J.M. (1990) *Touching the Rock*. London: Arrow Books.

Johnstone, D. (1991) Edward's alphabet. *Resurgence* No. 146: 34.

Kübler-Ross, E. (1969) *On Death and Dying*. London: Tavistock.

Kushner, H.S. (1986) *When All You've Ever Wanted Isn't Enough*. London: Pan Books.

Laurent, C. (1991) Right or wrong? *Nursing Times* **87** (45): 52–53.

Leavitt, F.J. (1996) Educating nurses for their future role in bioethics. *Nursing Ethics* **3** (1): 37–50.

Lewis, C.S. (1961) *A Grief Observed*. London: Faber and Faber.

Matthiesen, V. (1989) Guilt and grief: when daughters place mothers in nursing homes. *Journal of Gerontological Nursing* **15** (7): 11–15.

Maxwell, M. & Tschudin, V. (1990) *Seeing the Invisible; Modern Religious and Other Transcendent Experiences.* London: Arkana (Penguin).

Morse, J.M. & Carter, B.J. (1995) Strategies of enduring and the suffering of loss: modes of comfort used by a resilient survivor. *Holistic Nursing Practice* **9** (3): 38–52.

Oakley, A., McPherson, A. & Roberts, H. (1984) *Miscarriage* (rev. edn). London: Penguin.

Orona, C.J. (1990) Temporality and identity loss due to Alzheimer's Disease. *Social Science and Medicine* **30** (11): 1247–1256.

Oswin, M. (1991) *Am I Allowed to Cry? A Study of Bereavement Amongst People who have Learning Difficulties.* London: Souvenir Press.

Parkes, C.M. (1964) The effects of bereavement on physical and mental health; a study of the case records of widows. *British Medical Journal* **2**: 274–279.

Parkes, C.M. (1970) The first year of bereavement: a longitudinal study in the reaction of London widows to the death of their husbands. *Psychiatry* **33** (4): 444–467.

Parkes, C.M. (1971) Psycho-social transitions: a field for study. *Social Science and Medicine* **5**: 101–115.

Parkes, C.M. (1975a) *Bereavement: Studies of Grief in Adult Life.* Harmondsworth: Penguin.

Parkes, C.M. (1975b) The emotional impact of cancer of ear, nose and throat on patients and their families. *Journal of Laryngology and Otology* **89**: 1271–1275.

Patton, J.G. (1995) Looking for guarantees. *Holistic Nursing Practice* **9** (3): 4–10.

Payne, M. (1994) Mid-life loss and its consequences. *Changes* **12** (2): 132–135.

Penson, J. (1990) *Bereavement: A Guide for Nurses.* London: Harper and Row.

Rainey,H. (1990) Losses felt in later life. *Nursing Standard* **5** (8): 52–53.

Rando, T.A. (1984) *Grief, Dying and Death: Clinical Interventions for Caregivers.* Champaign, IL: Research Press.

Raphael, B. (1984) *The Anatomy of Bereavement: A Handbook for the Caring Professions.* London: Routledge.

Rhŷs-Evans, F. (1996) Head and neck cancer. Chapter 11, in Tschudin, V. (ed.) *Nursing the Patient with Cancer* (2nd edn). Hemel Hempstead: Prentice Hall.

Riggans, L. (1992) Living with loss. *Nursing Times* **88** (27): 34.

Rogers, C.R. (ed.) (1967) *The Therapeutic Relationship and Its Impact.* Madison: University of Wisconsin Press.

Rogers, C.R. (1980) *A Way of Being.* Boston, MA: Houghton Mifflin Co.

Rosen, H. (1986) *Unspoken Grief; Coping with Childhood Sibling Loss.* Lexington, MA: D.C. Heath & Co.

Schaefer, K.M. (1995) Women living in paradox: loss and discovery in chronic illness. *Holistic Nursing Practice* **9** (3): 63–74.

Schofield, I. (1995) Growth and development of the individual and family. Chapter 6, in Heath, H. (ed.) *Potter and Perry's Foundations in Nursing Theory and Practice.* London: Mosby.

Scott, P.A. (1995) Aristotle, nursing and health care ethics. *Nursing Ethics* **2** (4): 279–285.

Scrutton, S. (1989) *Counselling Older People: A Creative Response to Ageing*. London: Edward Arnold.

Seaver, A.M.H. (1994) My World Now. *Newsweek* June 27: 11.

Simmons, M. (1992) Helping children grieve. *Nursing Times* **88** (50): 30–32.

Speck, P. (1978) *Loss and Grief in Medicine*. London: Baillière Tindall.

Stewart, A. & Dent, A. (1994) *At a Loss; Bereavement Care When a Baby Dies*. London: Baillière Tindall.

Stone, J. (1980) Dissertation *On Bereavement*. Submitted to University of London, for Certificate in Student Counselling.

Thompson, J. (1987) Marriage. Chapter 5, in Virgo, L. (ed.) *First Aid in Pastoral Care*. Edinburgh: T & T Clark Ltd, pp. 55–67.

Tschudin, V. (1995) *Counselling Skills for Nurses* (4th edn). London: Baillière Tindall.

Ward, H. & Wild, J. (1995) *Guard the Chaos; Finding Meaning in Change*. London: Darton, Longman & Todd.

Weber, M. & Reimer, M. (1993) Laryngectomy: grieving disfigurement and dysfunction. *Canadian Nurse/Infirmière Canadienne* **89** (3): 31–34.

Wilson, M. (1995) *Dear Bryony*. London: Chester House Publications. (The author of the story on pp. 144–145 is untraced.)

Worden, J.W. (1991) *Grief Counselling and Grief Therapy: A Handbook for the Mental Health Practitioner* (2nd edn). London: Routledge.

Index
....